Palgrave Macmillan Studies in Family and Intimate Life

Series Editors
Graham Allan
Keele University, UK

Lynn Jamieson
University of Edinburgh, UK

David H.J. Morgan
University of Manchester, UK

The Palgrave Macmillan Studies in Family and Intimate Life series is impressive and contemporary in its themes and approaches' - Professor Deborah Chambers, Newcastle University, UK, and author of New Social Ties.

The remit of the Palgrave Macmillan Studies in Family and Intimate Life series is to publish major texts, monographs and edited collections focusing broadly on the sociological exploration of intimate relationships and family organization. The series covers a wide range of topics such as partnership, marriage, parenting, domestic arrangements, kinship, demographic change, intergenerational ties, life course transitions, step-families, gay and lesbian relationships, lone-parent households, and also non-familial intimate relationships such as friendships and includes works by leading figures in the field, in the UK and internationally, and aims to contribute to continue publishing influential and prize-winning research.

More information about this series at
http://www.springer.com/series/14676

Acknowledgements

The research that led to this book was made possible by a grant from the British Academy through their Small Grants scheme (BA Small Grant SG110141), and I am very grateful for that funding for enabling me to spend time, mostly during 2012, carrying out fieldwork. I should also like to thank everyone who took part in the interviews and focus groups for the study; the young parents, their partners and parents, and the members of staff, mostly in local authorities, who work with the young people. In particular, I should like to thank the youth workers in local authorities who agreed to take part and who helped to facilitate contacts with young people, and all at a time when they were going through reorganisations and restructuring of local government.

Thanks also to members of my study advisory group, Simon Forrest, Kate Guthrie, Sue Lewis, Jane McNaughton and Gail Teasdale.

Earlier versions of some sections of the book have been presented at a number of conferences: the British Sociological Association, the BSA Medical Sociology Group, the European Society for Health and Medical Sociology, and the International Qualitative Health Research conference. I was also asked to present findings at seminars at the Universities of Edinburgh, Glasgow, Central Lancashire, Leeds and Teesside. I am very grateful to friends and colleagues at those conferences and seminars who made insightful comments and asked questions that have undoubtedly helped me develop my thinking.

Although writing a book is a fairly solitary affair, I have been encouraged and supported by friends and colleagues, including my old ERDU colleagues Greg Rubin, Nicky Hall, Christina Dobson, Ingrid Ablett-Spence and Jackie Pankhurst, friends at Trevelyan College, Durham, especially Jon Warren, and many friends in the Medical Sociology world. Particular thanks go to Nicky Hall, Anna Tarrant, Ken Wallis and Margaret Wallis for reading and commenting on various sections and chapters. I should also like to thank Denis and Elizabeth Graves of Mocha in Richmond for the chocolate that has fuelled much of the writing.

I am very grateful to Professor David Morgan for his advice and encouragement during the writing and editing of the book. I am in no doubt that it is a better book for his support.

Finally, I thank my wonderful daughter Anna Feintuck, an inspiration herself, for her encouragement and unfailing support. I dedicate this book to her.

Contents

Editor's Introduction

Sociological enquiry frequently addresses the contrast between public perceptions and definitions of 'problems' and the way in which such problems are understood and experienced by the participants themselves. Studies of family and intimate life have provided several examples of this contrast and, in this present study, Sally Brown explores one of these: teenage pregnancy and parenting.

In terms of public perception and discussion, what is the nature of the 'problem' here? This study reminds us that it is no longer a question of the marital status of the mother that is at issue. It is, rather, a question of the youthfulness of the parents. Sally Brown presents the numerous concerns that converge in order to show how *teenage* motherhood has emerged as a problem in recent decades. It is bound up, she demonstrates, with issues of poverty and welfare and with understandings of cycles of disadvantage. But perhaps, at a deeper level, we are dealing with disruptions of normative temporal sequences. 'To every thing there is a season … A time to be born and a time to die …' (Ecclesiastes 3:1).

The author uses her sociological skills to present the construction of this particular problem in historical and comparative context. But her main concern, and the strength of this study, lies in the way in which she gets close to the stories of the women, and men, who are the focus of, but some distance from, these public debates. These stories are not 'bleak and depressing'. These young mothers are aware of the public stigma but reject it; a pregnancy may be unexpected or unplanned but it is by no means a disaster. It is a turning point and one which provides an opportunity for rewriting the life script, despite the local economic constraints.

One of the most impressive features of the study is the way that Sally Brown places these experiences in a wider family context. We are introduced to the wider networks of parents and grandparents, several of whom have, in the past, shared the experiences of the young mothers themselves. It 'kind of runs in the family'. Yet the public language of social pathology is replaced by a language of hope and aspiration. The young women continue to hope to continue their education and to get a good job while also planning to be a good mother. In many cases, the young fathers share in, and support, these aspirations. There is a mixture of realism and hope that runs through many of these stories and quotations that lie at the heart of this study.

In some ways this is a familiar story. The history of family life is full of accounts of departures from the normative sequencings. But there is a freshness in these accounts by young women and men, as well as by some professional practitioners, which encourages the reader to see these departures anew. And if some of our legislators have the opportunity to glance at these pages, then so much the better.

David H.J. Morgan
University of Manchester
Manchester, UK

Abbreviations

A level	Advanced level exams (exams usually taken at age 18 in England and Wales; grades determine university entrance)
AS level	Advanced Subsidiary level exams (the first component of an A level qualification)
CaSH	Contraception and Sexual Health
CCG	Clinical Commissioning Group
DfES	Department for Education and Skills
DH	Department of Health
DFLE	disability-free life expectancy
GCSE	General Certificate of Secondary Education (exams usually taken at age 16 in England and Wales)
ISD	Information Services Division (Scotland)
JSA	Jobseeker's Allowance
LE	life expectancy
NEET	Not in Education, Employment or Training
NHS	National Health Service
NVQ	National Vocational Qualification (exams taken in vocational/practical subjects in the UK, from age 17 and above)
ONS	Office for National Statistics (England and Wales)
PCT	Primary Care Trust
PSHE	Personal, Social and Health Education
SEU	Social Exclusion Unit

SRE   Sex and Relationships Education
TPIAG   Teenage Pregnancy Independent Advisory Group
TPS   Teenage Pregnancy Strategy
TPU   Teenage Pregnancy Unit

List of Figures

List of Tables

1

Introduction

Talking to a colleague at a research workshop, during the early days of the fieldwork for the study that is the subject of this book, the topic turned to the challenges of balancing work and childcare. Bea was in her late thirties, working part-time and writing up her PhD, and had two small children aged four and six. Sympathising with the challenges of having to manage home and school routines and somehow find time to write, I said that my daughter was five when I started my PhD. 'How old is she now?' Bea asked. 'Oh, she's 21, my PhD was a long time ago!' I said. 'You must have been really young when you had her.' 'No, I was 27.' 'But that *is* young!' she exclaimed. Around the same time, I met some of the young women who took part in one of the focus groups for the study. Chatting as we got settled, and telling them a little about myself, I mentioned that I had a daughter, aged 21. 'How many bairns has she got, then?' one of the young mothers asked. 'None,' I replied. 'She's at university.'

The same life story can look very different depending on the perspective of those viewing it. From Bea's perspective, 27 was early to have children, although the year I had my daughter, it was the average age for women having their first baby in the UK. Now, with over half of all births being to women over 30, I probably would seem young to many other

© The Editor(s) (if applicable) and The Author(s) 2016

S. Brown, *Teenage Pregnancy, Parenting and Intergenerational Relations,*
DOI 10.1057/978-1-137-49539-6_1

new mothers. On the other hand, for the young women I was talking to, all of whom had had babies during their teens, it seemed natural to assume that a 21-year-old would have had at least one child, although the teenage fertility rate was continuing to fall, so that only 3.4 per cent of all conceptions that year, in the UK, had been to teenagers. By the time the young women reach Bea's age, their oldest children will be adults, whereas Bea will be in her fifties before her children reach adulthood.

From an educational perspective, the various mothers' stories also illustrate very different, and classed, trajectories, with my daughter taking the middle-class route to adulthood, staying on at school and going to university at the 'right' age. Meanwhile, most of the young mums I spoke to had left school before they reached 18, some having been rare attenders from the age of 14 onwards. What Walkerdine et al. refer to as the 'terrible and central fact' (2001, p. 4) of the way social class divides working-class and middle-class girls is writ large on our lives.

> Don't panic, the teenage pregnancy epidemic is over!
> (*The Telegraph*, 28 February 2013)

> UK still has the highest rate of teen pregnancies in Western Europe
> (*Daily Mail*, 15 October 2014)

Stories about teenage pregnancy, and in particular the UK's record of having the highest teenage pregnancy rate in Europe, often feature in newspapers; the two headlines above are both written in response to announcements that the teenage pregnancy rate in the UK had fallen for both the years reported on in the stories, as it had been doing for several years previously, and as it has continued to do. In July 2015, as I was coming to the end of writing this book, the latest statistics on pregnancy and births in England and Wales were released, showing that once again, in 2014 there had been a decline in teenage pregnancy rates, to the lowest rate yet recorded. The report also notes that births to all age groups under 30 had fallen, and that the average age of mothers in England and Wales had crept over 30–30.2 in 2014 (ONS 2015). The most fertile age group in 2014 was women aged 30–34, and the under 20s had the largest decrease in fertility. Overall, birth rates fell for the second consecutive year, having risen for over a decade between 2001 and 2012. Almost half

(47.5 per cent) the babies born in 2014 were born outside marriage or civil partnership, compared to 42.4 per cent just ten years previously in 2004. Changing patterns of who has children and when, how families are formed and how people construct their family have changed dramatically over the past few decades.

NHS chief warns women not to wait until 30 to have baby as country faces a fertility timebomb
(*Daily Mail*, 30 May 2015)

Alongside the problematising of teenage pregnancy, stories in the popular press emerge fairly regularly about women 'leaving it too late', with the associated message that being a 'career woman' will lead to having regrets at lost opportunities to become a mother. The shift in fertility patterns has led some newspapers to argue that young and poorly educated women are having too many babies while clever women are not having enough, if they are having any at all. In the summer of 2012, Dr Lucy Worsley, Chief Curator at Historic Royal Palaces and well-known presenter of historical documentaries on the BBC, talked about the connections between her educational path and not having children, saying that she had been 'educated out of the reproductive function'. When this led to media stories about some women feeling 'too clever' to have children, Dr Worsley explained that rather than it being an issue of cleverness, it was more about the strong emphasis that her school had placed on becoming educated to as high a level as possible, which left little time for women in her situation to think about having a family (Wintle 2013). The flurry of media interest led the *Daily Mail* to link supposedly high numbers of teenage mothers with falling numbers of intelligent mothers, and claim that the wrong type of women were having children.

Both younger and older mothers are positioned by the media as making wrong choices in terms of timing (Hadfield et al. 2007), the younger ones because they are perceived to be too young to cope, the older ones because they may need treatment for infertility having left it too late to try to conceive (Macvarish 2010; Perrier 2013). Poor parenting, in particular single parenting, has also been blamed for a range of social problems, including riots in the UK in summer 2011, prompting Sarah

Teather, then Children's Minister, to announce the piloting of parenting lessons in three areas of the UK in 2012, saying 'it is the government's moral and social duty to make sure we support all parents at this critical time' (Teather 2011). Although not compulsory, and not aimed solely at young or single parents, it is an example of a technical, and individualised, solution to the 'problem' of poor parenting, which could easily be used as an instrument of blame: if your child turns out 'bad' it is your fault for not attending parenting classes. As an individualised solution, it does not address structural or educational disadvantage, and it is ironic that the classes were announced while funding for Sure Start (a measure aimed at addressing disadvantage, particularly in early years' education) was no longer ring fenced, with the effect that many local authorities in the UK were cutting service provision. This is a shift of parenting support from being part of welfare services to being the subject of individualised corrective measures. Structural inequalities are rewritten as a set of factors that put young people at risk, and individualism means that people are responsible for their own fate; thus young people are 'at risk' not because of class or circumstance, but as a result of their own irrational behaviour. Furthermore, there is a sense in which young parents are criticised for not making the 'right' choices, but those choices, and life courses more generally, are overwhelmingly determined by middle-class norms and choices.

It sometimes seems, then, as though women are continually bombarded with advice, instruction and criticism as far as motherhood is concerned: don't have babies too soon, don't leave it too late; to be childless is to be pitied, to have too many is to be vilified. Once the baby is born, will the mother be a Yummy Mummy, a Tiger Mom, Alpha Mum or Pramface? Will they become a 'Problem Family', faced with interventions and sanctions for not being the right type of family? It seems not only that the ideal window in which a woman can become a mother is narrowing, but also that how to be an acceptable mother is increasingly constrained.

The Generations Study

In the chapters that follow, the issues raised in this introduction will be drawn out as part of the discussion of the findings from 'The Generations Study'. This was a British Academy funded study about families where more than one generation had been a teenage mother, the intention being to explore how decisions were made in those families about when (or whether) to become a parent, and what differences and similarities there might be in the experiences of the generations across time. One key question was what role, if any, the older generation had in influencing the decisions of the younger one about becoming a teenage mother. In part, this was an exploration of whether there is any truth in the notion of underclass theorists such as Charles Murray (Murray 1990) that there is a transmission from one generation to another of a range of aspects of deprivation, thus perpetuating those cycles of disadvantage. Another angle on the same question was to explore whether there were aspects of local cultures, in other words influences beyond individual families, that meant certain local authorities in the UK regularly appeared towards the top of 'league tables' of teenage pregnancy rates. In other words, is it something that runs in families? Is it something that happens 'round here'? And if so, why?

Chapter 2 begins by setting out the history of problematic motherhood, from the moral problems of illegitimacy and unmarried mothers, through lone parents, and finally to the appearance of teenage mothers as a social problem to be solved. The chapter discusses the policy approaches adopted over time, from an initial public health approach focussing on the well-being of the children, to a more recent argument encompassing the likely poor health of mother and child. This chapter also discusses international comparisons of teenage pregnancy, setting the UK in the context of European experience as well as the 'Anglophone nations' (Chandola et al. 2002) of Australia, Canada, New Zealand and the USA.

In Chapter 3, the settings where the fieldwork for 'The Generations Study' took place are introduced in order to illustrate the cultural, social and economic contexts within which the participants live. The inspiration for the study itself provides part of the background, and the chapter also sets out the theoretical frameworks that informed the study and the analysis.

Chapters 4 to 8 are the heart of the book, where we hear the participants tell their stories. The chapters take a chronological approach from becoming pregnant (in Chap. 4) and being a parent (in Chap. 5), while Chapter 6 explores how the young parents and their new baby sit within the family, both the new one they have created, and their wider networks of grandparents, siblings, aunts and uncles. Chapter 7 focusses on the people who work with young parents in healthcare and welfare settings, and considers their views and accumulated knowledge about the local contexts within which they work. Chapter 8 looks to the future for the young parents, and discusses the aims and aspirations they have for themselves and their children.

In the concluding chapter, I discuss constructions of parenthood and motherhood in social, cultural and policy contexts, and explore the interactions between the individual biographies of the participants in the study and the familial and social settings and cultures in which they live. I introduce the concept of 'rewriting the life script', an active process which young people undertake to make sense of themselves and their lives as parents. Finally I look to potential future policy developments which may impact upon the lives of young parents.

References

Chase-Lansdale, P. L., Brooks-Gunn, J., & Zamsky, E. S. (1994). Young African-American multigenerational families in poverty: Quality of mothering and grandmothering. *Child Development, 65*(2), 373–393.

Hadfield, L. Rudoe, N. and Sanderson-mann, J. (2007). Motherhood, choice and the British media: Time to reflect. *Gender and Education, 19*(2), 255–263.

Macvarish, J. (2010). The effect of 'risk-thinking' on the contemporary construction of teenage motherhood. *Health, Risk & Society, 12*(4), 313–322.

Murray, C. (1990). *The emerging British underclass*. London: IEA.

Office for National Statistics. (2015). *Statistical bulletin: Births in England and Wales 2013*. London: Stationery Office.

Perrier, M. (2013). No right time: The significance of reproductive timing for younger and older mothers' moralities. *The Sociological Review, 61*(1), 69–87.

Taulbut, M., Walsh, D., Parcell, S., Hanlon, P., Hartmann, A., Poirier, G., et al. (2011). *Health and its determinants in Scotland and other parts of post-industrial Europe: The 'Aftershock of Deindustrialisation' study – phase 2*. Glasgow: Glasgow Centre for Population Health.

Walkerdine, V., Lucey, H., & Melody, J. (2001). *Growing-up girl: Psycho-social explorations of gender and class*. London: Palgrave.

Wintle, A. (2013). Lucy Worsley: My family values. *The Guardian*, Retrieved from http://www.theguardian.com/lifeandstyle/2013/apr/12/lucy-worsley-my-family-values

2

'They're Not This Kind of Thing That You Think They Are': Patterns, Trends and Policy

In many Western nations, such as Australia, Canada, New Zealand, the UK and the USA, teenage pregnancy and parenting have been a recurring concern for policymakers, politicians and the media, as well as for professionals in the fields of public health and social welfare. Although the motives for each sector may differ in terms of their reasons for concern, the effect is the same: to keep the issue high on policy and public agendas. In the UK, successive governments have defined teenage pregnancy as a problem that needs addressing, although the definition of the nature of the problem has varied. However, as Wilson and Huntington (2006) pointed out, this policy agenda has coincided with declining teenage birth rates in almost all Western developed nations. This chapter examines the data and explores the development of policies concerned with teenage pregnancy and parenting. It also considers the pictures painted by the media, and the relationship between media presentations of a problem and political approaches to solving it. The focus will be mainly on the UK, with international comparisons drawn where data allow. I begin by setting out a history of how some types of mothers have been regarded as problems, and the shift from viewing problematic motherhood as an issue of morality to a concern for public health and social policy.

© The Editor(s) (if applicable) and The Author(s) 2016   **7**
S. Brown, *Teenage Pregnancy, Parenting and Intergenerational Relations*,
DOI 10.1057/978-1-137-49539-6_2

Problematic Motherhood

Differing aspects of motherhood, or the form that motherhood takes, have been regarded as problematic for very many decades. At various times from the nineteenth century onwards, unmarried, single and teenage mothers have been regarded as morally or socially unacceptable, although the age of the mother was less problematic than her marital status for much of the twentieth century.

Illegitimacy

In the nineteenth and early twentieth centuries, illegitimacy was a major concern in the UK and elsewhere. In cases where a couple conceived a baby prior to marriage, the problem was avoided by the couple getting married before the baby was born, thus ensuring legitimacy. Age was, at this point in time, irrelevant in terms of whether or not the conception and the subsequent child were acceptable, the overarching issue being a moral one regarding marriage. The ramifications of the 'stain of illegitimacy', as described by Jane Austen in *Emma*, published in 1816, proved a rich source of inspiration for novelists such as Dickens, Trollope, Austen and Gaskell as they charted social life and social change throughout the nineteenth century. At that point in time, the problem was perceived not only as one of low morals in the mother; the child was also believed to have a flawed character.

In situations where the pregnant woman could not marry the father of her child, she was often seen as bringing disgrace upon herself and her family. Often sent away to give birth in secret, she would return home alone having had the child adopted, never to be spoken of again. Mother and baby homes were set up for this purpose, often by voluntary bodies such as churches. In some cases a pregnancy resulted in the woman, but not the man, effectively being punished for having sex. In Ireland, this resulted in the scandal of the Magdalene Laundries, homes run by the Catholic Church for 'fallen women', captured memorably and shockingly in the film *The Magdalene Sisters*, written and directed in 2002 by Peter Mullan. The film was based on a book charting experiences of four women in a Dublin Magdalene Laundry between 1964 and 1968. In the UK and the USA, women could be institutionalised in the large asylums dating from Victorian times. One of the shocking aspects of the move to community care and the closing of those institutions in the UK in the 1970s and 1980s was the way it revealed how many elderly women were in such places as a result of having had a child as an unmarried mother in the 1920s and 1930s. As highlighted by the 2013 film *Philomena*, directed by Stephen Frears, based on the book *The Lost Child of Philomena Lee* by journalist Martin Sixsmith (2009), most of these women, both in the Laundries and in asylums, will have given their children up for adoption, many unwillingly.

Shifting Attitudes Towards Lone Mothers

While the status of unmarried mothers remained shameful in many minds throughout the first half of the twentieth century, the position changed after the Second World War. Thane and Evans (2012) suggest that this shift had in fact begun during the First World War, when state support had been given to the 'unmarried wives' and illegitimate children of servicemen, although lone mothers, as opposed to cohabiting but unmarried ones, were not supported. Their book is a history of The National Council for the Unmarried Mother and her Child, which changed its name to National Council for One Parent Families in 1973 and is now known as Gingerbread. The council was established in 1918, in part as a response to concerns that the death rate for illegitimate children was higher than that of legitimate ones, and as such can be seen as one of a range of responses, from both state and voluntary sectors, to deal with perceived threats to the state in the form of the poor health and well-being of the population. The roots of the welfare state as a whole can of course be traced back to the discovery that high numbers of those volunteering at the time of recruitment for the Boer War (1899–1902) failed army entrance tests due to being medically unfit. This will not be the last time that we see the poor health of children being used to justify interventions in family life.

Thane and Evans argue that by the time of the Second World War, illegitimacy was becoming less secretive, and attitudes were shifting. Lone motherhood was also not uncommon, not least due to the numbers of women who were widowed due to the war, while the creation of the welfare state benefitted all mothers. The National Assistance Act of 1948 gave unmarried mothers the same assistance as those who were married, unlike earlier forms of social assistance which had helped widows but excluded divorced and unmarried mothers.

Despite this shift, single women were still 'sent away' to have their babies in mother and baby homes, with adoption still seen as the ideal solution if a 'shotgun marriage' was not an option, and this approach persisted into the 1960s. In 1966 in England and Wales, for example, there were 172 mother and baby homes, 148 of which were run by voluntary organisations and 24 by local authorities (Thane and Evans 2012). The 1960s were heralded as a time of massive social change, not least in the realms of sexual behaviour, partly because of the discovery of 'the pill', although a number of commentators have suggested that this change was neither massive nor evenly spread. Nevertheless, by 1972 there were only 65 homes, which the National Council for One Parent Families believed was partly due to women feeling able to stay in their communities, due to changing attitudes towards illegitimacy.

Marriage and Cohabitation

The 1970s was a period when attitudes to marriage also changed, while the age of the mother had not yet registered as a major concern. This is captured in Alan Johnson's moving and powerful memoir *Please, Mr Postman*. In one passage he describes how when he and his wife Judy moved to a new area in 1969, when he was 19 and she was 23, they fudged the dates of their marriage, as Judy already had a daughter, and they did not want their new neighbours to know that he was not the father of one of his children. That they were 17 and 21 when they got married, with one child already and another on the way, was not the issue; that Judy had been an unmarried mother was. By 1975, when he adopted the older girl, which involved the neighbours being interviewed and the truth about their backstory emerging, attitudes had changed enough for him to be able to write 'In the event, it didn't matter; none of our neighbours even mentioned it and I very much doubt by then that it would have been the subject of scurrilous gossip' (Johnson 2014, p. 179), which it may well have been in 1969.

During the 1960s and 1970s, cohabitation became much more popular as marriage became less popular, in both the UK and the USA. Furstenberg (2007) explains the seeming contradiction in the data whereby the number of unmarried teenage mothers in the USA rose during the 1960s while the teenage pregnancy rate fell; fewer young women became pregnant, and many of those that did chose not to get married, so although there were more unmarried mothers, the teenage birth rate was falling. In fact, the same applies to older women, who were also less likely to marry than in previous decades. With the rise in cohabitation, condemnation of unmarried mothers lessened. More teenage mothers also kept their babies, rather than giving them up for adoption. In 1971 in the UK, three-quarters of births to teens occurred within marriage, although conception may have taken place prior to the wedding (Arai 2009), and around 20 per cent of babies born to teenagers were adopted (Duncan et al. 2010). By 2004, only 10 per cent of births to teens in the UK were to teenagers who were married (Arai 2009), although 30 per cent were cohabiting, and another quarter registered the birth jointly although with the parents living at separate addresses (Duncan et al. 2010). The changes in patterns of teenage relationships demonstrated by these figures reflect patterns in older age groups, and these changes in the way families were constituted were seen across the population as a whole.

The Emergence of Teenage Motherhood as a Problem

While the focus remained on the marital status of mothers, and on lone motherhood, there was little direct attention in terms of policy apart from welfare support. Teenage motherhood as a separate issue from lone motherhood was not the focus of policy in either the USA or the UK. Arai (2009) identifies the shift in concern from marital status to age of mother as occurring in the late 1960s to early 1970s in the USA, but not until later in the UK. The first significant appearance of teenagers as a policy focus, in terms of UK government policies, occurred in the early 1990s in the context of health policy. In terms of health outcomes, it is widely thought that pregnancy is a risk to both teenage mother and her baby, which provides a public health rationale for trying to prevent teenage pregnancy. Although the picture is complex, it appears that first teenage births are less at risk of stillbirth or prematurity than those of older women, and have a lower risk of delivery by emergency caesarean section (Smith and Pell 2001; Jivraj et al. 2010). Some studies (Fraser et al. 1995; Olausson et al. 1999) that have shown an increased risk for maternal death, preterm delivery and low birthweight have not controlled for maternal smoking, which is one of the highest risk factors for those outcomes, and teenage mothers are much more likely to smoke than older mothers.

The Conservative governments of 1979–1997 placed the reduction of teenage pregnancy rates in the remit of the National Health Service (NHS), with targets being included in the *Health of the Nation* White Paper (Department of Health 1992). This set out five target areas, of which sexual health was one, although at that point in time, there was a greater emphasis on sexually transmitted diseases than on teenage pregnancy, not least because of the prominence of HIV/AIDS in the public consciousness. As Baroness Cumberlege stated on introducing the White Paper in the House of Lords, 'AIDS is the most significant new threat to public health this century. In improving sexual health generally lies the greatest scope for preventing HIV infection and the spread of that terrible disease' (Hansard 1992). Although teenage pregnancy featured in the targets, it related to conceptions to under 16-year-olds only; 16-year-olds and upwards were not mentioned. The target was to reduce conceptions in under 16-year-olds by at least 50 per cent from 9.5 per 1000 13–15 year-olds (the rate in 1989) to no more than 4.8 by 2000. However, *Health of the Nation* targets did not always take precedence for local health authorities faced with continually changing priorities from the Department of Health, such as targets for the reduction of waiting lists, and as a result, targets in the five key areas were not reached (University of Leeds et al. 1998), including those for teenage conceptions (ONS 1998).

Labour's Teenage Pregnancy Strategy

The Labour government elected in 1997 made reduction of teenage pregnancy a high priority, and in 1999 published the Teenage Pregnancy Report (SEU 1999) and launched the Teenage Pregnancy Strategy (TPS). Like the previous government, the aim was to reduce teenage pregnancies by half; however, whereas the previous target related to under 16-year-olds, the targets in the TPS included under 18-year-olds. The expansion of the problem age group, from under 16, to under 18, is worth noting. As Macvarish argues, 'not only did this instantly inflate the perceived problem, it also redefined it' (Macvarish 2010, p. 317). She suggests that this made the problem one of young women having children, rather than the problem being unwanted conceptions, as older teenagers are more likely to continue with an unplanned pregnancy while younger ones are more likely to have a termination. Although there is a moral overtone to the TPS (Carabine 2007), this was the first clear shift away from the overt moralising about marriage that characterised the history of problematic motherhood to that point, and towards problematising motherhood based on age.

A section of the report which sets out why teenage pregnancy matters as a problem opens with a list of health and welfare problems connected to teenage pregnancy: 'Teenage parents tend to have poor ante-natal health, lower birth weight babies and higher infant mortality rates. Their own health and their children's is worse than average' (SEU 1999, p. 23). Thus the connection between age and poor health became a major reason for policy intervention. The increasing emphasis on the likely poor health of children as a result of their mothers' age is also an echo of the very early moves to introduce social welfare in the UK in the early twentieth century, where the poor health firstly of military recruits and later of illegitimate children became reasons for intervention by the state.

Locating teenage pregnancy within the Social Exclusion Unit (SEU), as opposed to the Department of Health, was an indicator of the significance of social exclusion as a concept and policy driver across a broad spectrum of government activity for the new Labour government. However, despite the identification of teenage pregnancy as a social problem, and the connection to social exclusion and deprivation, poverty, low educational achievement and poor employment opportunities, the measures to reduce rates were individualistic and behaviouralist, which Arai labels 'technical/educational' (2009, p. 64). Here, the focus was on providing information (through improved sex and relationship education) which would enable teenagers to correctly use the technical means of avoiding pregnancy now widely available; that is, it was based on an assumption that unplanned pregnancies could be completely avoided by the correct use of contraception.

The other aspect of the TPS was to encourage behaviour change in order to enable teenagers to manage their risks and behave as economically rational beings, thereby avoiding pregnancy, and thus avoiding social exclusion (Duncan 2007; Hoggart 2012). Social exclusion as a concept is poorly defined, although for the purposes of the TPS, the SEU's description is illustrative: it is 'a shorthand term for what happens when people or areas suffer from a combination of linked problems such as unemployment, discrimination, poor skills, low incomes, poor housing, high crime, bad health and family breakdown' (SEU 2004). This is a different approach to previous attempts to reduce health inequalities, which tended to focus on the individual, as in the *Health of the Nation* targets around behaviour and lifestyle. This approach identifies individuals but also the place-based nature of some types of disadvantage. As far as teenage pregnancy is concerned, this was taken forward by identifying 'hotspots', which were areas experiencing the highest teenage pregnancy rates; hotspots as a concept first appear in the TPS in 1999, and are referenced again in the 2006 *Next Steps* progress report (DfES 2006a), which highlighted the different speed at which local authorities were moving towards the 2010 targets. The focus on economic participation in the form of employment, or preparation for employment, as a way of getting out of social exclusion can also be seen in the introduction of the concept of the young person who was a 'NEET', which was shorthand for those not in education, employment or training. As well as attempting to reduce the rates of teenage pregnancy, the TPS had an explicit target to increase the numbers of teenage parents in education, training or employment to 60 per cent by 2010; by ensuring fewer young parents were NEETs, this would reduce social exclusion.

However, these arguments about social exclusion assume that the teenagers concerned were socially included to begin with, and would become excluded as a result of a pregnancy. The packaging of teenage pregnancy with policies to tackle the issue of NEETs also makes assumptions about the form of exclusion being one of economic exclusion, and therefore capable of solution by ensuring that young parents are in employment, or in training to become employed.

A key point to note about the launch of the TPS was its timing in relation to trends in birth rates. At the time when Prime Minister Tony Blair made his famous remarks about 'shattered lives and blighted futures' in the foreword to the report (SEU 1999, p. 4), teenage pregnancy rates were roughly the same as they had been in the 1950s; there had been a steady decline from a high of 50.6 births per 1000 women under 20 in 1971 to 30.9 per 1000 in 1999 (ONS 2006). Conception rates for women under 18 and girls under 16 show a similar decline. As Fig. 2.1 shows, the birth rate was also falling for women in their twenties, and increasing for women aged 30 and over, reflected in a shift from the average age of mother at first birth from 23 in the late 1960s, to 30 in 2013, the first time it reached 30 in the UK (ONS 2014a). A similar pattern has occurred in other developed countries (United Nations 2003) such as Canada (Statistics Canada 2013b).

One consequence of the increase in the average age at which women have their first child is that if there is a larger proportion of older mothers in the population, and it becomes a perceived norm that women wait longer before having children, then teenage mothers become more visible and appear to be a demographic anomaly. Whitley and Kirmayer (2008), in their Canadian study, found that mothers in their early twenties felt that they were experiencing the stigma and judgemental attitudes that teenage mothers received, partly as a result of the increase in average age at first birth in Canada to 28 (in 2003), with about half of first births being to mothers aged over 30.

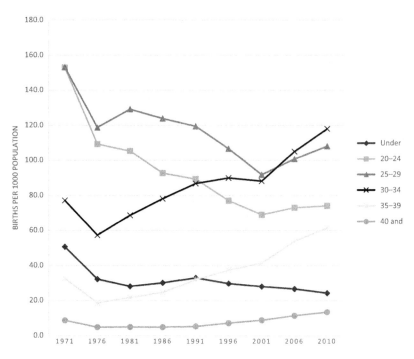

Fig. 2.1   Age specific fertility rates, 1971–2010, England and Wales. *Source*: ONS 2011

As Arai discusses in her comprehensive review of New Labour's approach to teenage pregnancy and parenting policies (Arai 2009), the TPS was a clear break from earlier approaches to reducing teenage pregnancy, marking a move away from seeing it as a moral problem to its reconstitution as a social problem. There was also a much more explicit acknowledgement that poverty and deprivation played a part in health inequalities, of which teenage pregnancy was seen to be a part, than had been accepted by previous Conservative governments.

The key targets set in the TPS were to halve the under-18 conception rate by 2010, and to establish a downward trend in the under-16 rate, with a further target of increasing the number of teenage parents in education, training or employment to 60 per cent also with a 2010 date. In May 2010, a general election in the UK resulted in the Labour Party leaving office to be replaced by a Coalition government formed by the Conservative Party and the Liberal Democrats. Before examining their approach to teenage pregnancy and parenting, it is worth considering the extent to which the TPS had been a success (or not), and hence the legacy left by such a concerted effort on the part of a UK government to focus on one specific aspect of social policy.

Did the Strategy Work?

Two reviews published during the life of the strategy had found that teenage pregnancies were falling in the UK, although due to the relatively short time periods being evaluated, the extent to which the measures implemented under the auspices of the strategy were a direct cause of the reduction was unclear. A report commissioned by the Teenage Pregnancy Support Unit (Wellings et al. 2005) suggested that as the rate of decline was steepest in areas that received more funding to implement the strategy, the targeting of funding at the most deprived areas had worked well. However, it had not been possible to link a decrease in conceptions to specific strategy-related activities at a local level, although as the authors point out, the latest conception data available to them dated from 2002, just two years into the strategy. In *Teenage Pregnancy: Accelerating the Strategy to 2010* (DfES 2006b) it was acknowledged that progress towards the 2010 targets had been uneven, with some local authorities, such as City of Westminster, experiencing a steep decline, whilst others saw almost no change, and some, such as Barking and Dagenham, had a significant increase (31.5 per cent between 1998 and 2004). It was clear at this point, almost half way into the time period for the strategy, that although some local authorities might meet their targets, the overall national target of a halving of the under-18 conception rate would not be met. Arai (2009) suggests that the reasons for this could include having unrealistic initial targets that could never have been achieved over one decade, uneven implementation of the strategy, or simply that the strategy was inappropriate for some areas. What was also clear from *Accelerating the Strategy*, she suggests, is that the authors could not definitively account for the changes in rates. While Arai refers to 'a barely concealed naming and shaming' (2009,

p. 69), the list of poorly performing local authorities in Annex 1 of the report means they are not concealed at all. The report seems to imply that reduction in teenage pregnancy rates was linked to how well the strategy had been implemented at local level, when it states that 'high performing areas have demonstrated that if the strategy is implemented effectively and with strong commitment, teenage conception rates can fall very substantially' (DfES 2006b, p. 15). The implication that areas that had not reached their targets were performing poorly because of a lack of commitment by local staff led to resentment on the part of some local Teenage Pregnancy Coordinators (personal communication), who felt that they and their staff were being blamed for failing to hit targets when some aspects of the challenges of reducing teenage pregnancy were outside their control, and that insufficient attention was being paid by the Department of Education and Skills (DfES) to specific local circumstances. Despite the acknowledgement in the TPS that poverty and deprivation played a part in teenage pregnancy, local teenage pregnancy coordinators were expected to hit targets without the means to affect wider social contexts.

Other studies found that teenage pregnancy rates were falling, and debated why. Wilkinson et al. (2006) compared a period prior to the strategy (1994–1998) with the first few years of its existence (1999–2003) and reported that under-18 conception rates had fallen by an average of 2 per cent per year between 1998 and 2003, whilst noting that this was below the rate needed to achieve the 2010 target. The net changes between 1994–1998 and 1999–2003 were a 3.2 per cent fall in conceptions amongst women aged 15–17 years (1.4 per 1000 women), a 7.5 per cent rise in abortions, and a 10.6 per cent fall in births. They argue that the 'evidence that the declines have been greatest in areas receiving higher amounts of strategy-related funding provides limited evidence of the effect of England's national teenage pregnancy strategy' (Wilkinson et al. 2006, p. 1879). However, in a commentary in the same issue of *The Lancet*, Galavotti and Green (2006) were not convinced that the decline in rates, which they argued was only small, was due to the success of the strategy. Other commentators felt the same when, in 2009, data from 2007 were released showing that teenage pregnancy rates had increased that year in both the under-16 and under-18 age groups (O'Hara 2009). The Guardian cited several commentators referring to the rise as a 'blip', and linked the rise in rates to a story the same month about a 13-year-old boy getting his 15-year-old girlfriend pregnant. *The Times* newspaper responded to the news that rates had increased by calling the TPS a policy disaster (Arai 2009, p. 70). Duncan et al. (2010) demonstrate how newspapers persist in presenting atypical cases as commonplace, and then make connections between teenage parents and the moral breakdown of British society. Arai (2009) notes the sensational, salacious and overwhelmingly negative tone of newspaper stories about teenage pregnancy, while Hadfield et al. (2007) highlight the vilification of teenage mothers by the tabloid press. That the *Daily Mail*, as quoted in the introduction, could report the lowest ever teenage pregnancy rates (in 2014) with a headline stating that they were the highest in Europe, rather than highlighting the steep decline, seems to confirm a continual search for negativity on the part of some of the press as far as teenage pregnancy is concerned.

In December 2010 the Teenage Pregnancy Independent Advisory Group (TPIAG) published their final report (TPIAG 2010). TPIAG had been established in 2000 to advise ministers on the implementation and development of the TPS, and to monitor progress towards achievement of the targets. In their view, the strategy had been a success, even though there had been some disappointing elements. They reported that the under-18 conception rate had fallen by 13 per cent between 1998 and 2008, and the birth rate for that group had fallen by 25 per cent over the same period. Their view for the shortfall, in terms of the 50 per cent target, was that this had been too ambitious a target for a relatively short timescale of ten years, particularly given that teenage pregnancy and poverty were closely interlinked. However, despite acknowledging that poverty was a key influence on rates, and therefore teenage pregnancy was unlikely to be reduced unless measures to reduce poverty were implemented at the same time, they went on to say that as some local authorities had reduced their under-18 conception rates by up to 45 per cent from the 1998 base line, this 'proved the strategy worked when it was applied properly'. Conversely, 'some local areas failed to implement the strategy effectively and as a consequence their teenage pregnancy rate stayed high—or in some cases increased' (TPIAG 2010, p. 1). It appears, then, that once again local authorities were being blamed for failures even when the magnitude of some factors out of their control was being acknowledged.

By the time the TPIAG produced their report, it had become clear that the Coalition government were embarking on severe cuts to a wide range of public sector programmes across health and welfare, including major reforms of the NHS, and a reduction in local authority budgets. The group expressed their concern that the absence of the clear leadership on teenage pregnancy that the TPS had provided would result in the loss of a coordinated approach between local authorities and the NHS. They described it as '*truly shocking* (my emphasis) to hear about the current level of disinvestment, the loss of posts and projects and closure of CaSH (Contraception and Sexual Health) services' (TPIAG 2010, p. 2) which is unusually strong criticism of government from an advisory body. Indeed, it would appear that the abolition of Primary Care Trusts (PCTs) and their replacement by much smaller Clinical Commissioning Groups (CCGs) has led to a loss of coordinated services across some local authorities, who find that rather than having one PCT to deal with, they may have up to six CCGs covering the same area.

The TPIAG commented that there had been a 'significant and positive' culture change in the way that young people, their parents, and their schools talked about sex and relationships, and approached sex education. They welcomed the Schools White Paper (DfE 2010) which promised a review of the curriculum in maintained schools, but expressed regret that Personal, Social and Health Education (PSHE) and Sex and Relationships Education (SRE) would not be included in the review. In fact, later efforts to make sex education, including topics such as relationships and consent, compulsory in UK schools failed to be accepted by parliament (BBC Democracy Live 2014; Hansard 2014). It remains the case that in England and Wales, sex education remains part of the science curriculum, academies and free schools are not obliged to follow the national curriculum, and parents can withdraw their children from sex education lessons in any school.

Once the 2010 data became available, it was clear that the results of the strategy were mixed. A clear downward trend in the number of births to under 16-year-olds had been established, but the target of halving the numbers of births to under 18-year-olds had not been met, although the rate of teenage conceptions in England and Wales was at its lowest in 2010 since 1969, which is when comparable data first started being collected by the Office for National Statistics (ONS). An increase in the rate in 2006/2007 appeared to have been a blip, as the downward trend was re-established in 2008. There do not appear to be any explanations for the rise, but the same blip in the overall downward trend also occurred in the USA for the same time period (CDC 2007). In his review of data for the time period covering the whole of TPS's existence, Conrad (2012) found that although under-18 conception rates fell between 1998 and 2010, rates of deprivation-based inequalities between local authorities did not change, with a clear link between deprivation and under-18 conception rates.

The Coalition government's NHS reforms included the removal of public health services from the NHS, and the return of the public health function to local authorities, who had had that responsibility until 1974. Since April 2013, when they assumed their new roles, local authorities have had responsibility for commissioning provision of contraceptive services, apart from the services provided by GPs, and also services for some sexually transmitted infections, although HIV services remain with the NHS, as does commissioning for abortion services. Although the inclusion of a target for the reduction of teenage pregnancy rates in the *Public Health Outcomes Framework* (Department of Health 2013a) means that it is a policy area that will still need attention, it seems likely that the fragmentation of commissioning for sexual health services and the shift away from explicit policies and leadership focussing on teenage pregnancy will result in poorer coordination across local authorities and health services. As the coordinated response was seen as a hallmark of the TPS, it remains to be seen whether we will see changes in rates of teenage pregnancy alongside these organisational changes. It could be argued that if teenage pregnancy rates continue to fall despite the organisational changes, this is an indication that the structures and strategies put in place had not themselves caused the decline; as the downward trend was clear even before 1999, a continuation of it may just be what would have happened anyway.

Data published by the ONS (ONS 2014a) in early 2014 showed that the under-18 conception rate in England had fallen to its lowest point yet recorded, with a reduction of 41 per cent between 1998 and 2012. Hadley argues that 'this significant decline is the result of the previous government's 10-year TPS and the concerted effort of local government, health organisations, services and frontline practitioners' (2014, p. 44) while pointing out that the strategy's original target of a 50 per cent reduction in conceptions had not yet been reached. The latest data available at the time of writing (summer 2015) were released by the ONS in February 2015 (ONS 2015) and relate to 2013; these show that the under-18 conception rate for 2013 was the lowest since 1969, and that there had been a fall of 13 per cent in the under-18 rate and 14 per cent in the under-16 rate between 2012 and 2013. It is interesting to note that for the population as a whole, conception rates in 2013 increased for women aged 35 years and over, and decreased for women aged under 35 years, compared to the previous year. This suggests that the average age of mothers at first birth may continue to increase to beyond 30, making teenage mothers even more of a demographic anomaly.

International Comparisons

One of the reasons given for concern at the rate of teenage pregnancy in the UK is that it is high compared to other countries, particularly those in Western Europe. The most comprehensive review of teenage fertility currently available remains the UNICEF report of 2001 on teenage births in rich nations, which showed that in 1998 the USA had the highest birth rate for teenagers at 52 per 1000 women aged 15–19, the UK had a rate of 30.8, which was the highest in Europe, with Switzerland at 5.5 per 1000 the lowest in Europe. The Netherlands, often held up as an example of good practice as far as sex education is concerned, had a rate of 6.2 per 1000. Three-quarters of the total number of births were in what the authors labelled the five anglophone countries (UK, USA, Australia, Canada and New Zealand), and while they emphasise the complexity of reasons for different rates across all the countries in the report, they suggest that the inclusiveness of society, as measured by income inequality and teenagers remaining in education, may be a factor. New Zealand, the USA and the UK, all in the top six as far as rates are concerned, are also the least inclusive societies with the highest degrees of income inequality (UNICEF 2001).

It has been suggested that there is an 'Anglo-Saxon domination of teenage pregnancy' (Arai 2009, p. 9) based on international comparisons of teenage pregnancy and fertility rates (Chandola et al. 2002) which place the USA, UK, Canada, Australia and New Zealand at the top of tables comparing rates in developed nations, such as the data produced by UNICEF. However, as Table 2.1 shows, although these countries are often regarded as comparable, Canada and Australia have rates significantly lower than the other three countries. A comparison of England and Wales, Canada and the USA found that between 1996 and 2006 teenage pregnancy rates declined in each of those countries, although rates in England and Wales and the USA remain consistently higher than in Canada (McKay and Barrett 2010).

Chandola et al. (2002) suggest that as part of the English-speaking world, these five anglophone nations have several historical, cultural and demographic characteristics in common, largely to do with patterns of migration, education and employment, that contribute to their similar fertility patterns, in particular a 'hump' in births before the age of 25 that is not seen in European countries. While there is a trend in later births across all developed countries, the shift in patterns has been more

Table 2.1 Teenage birth rates per 1000 population in five anglophone countries, 1999 and 2013

	Teenage birth rates	
	1999	2013
Australia	18.1	14.6
Canada	18.6	12.6*
New Zealand	28.9	21.5
USA	48.8	26.5
England and Wales	45.1	24.5
Scotland	43.2	24.5

Source: ONS (2014a), ISD (2015), Statistics Canada (2013a, 2013b), Statistics New Zealand (2014), Australian Bureau of Statistics (2014), Department of Health and Human Services, Office of Adolescent Health (2015)
*This figure is for 2011

uniform in continental European countries than in the anglophone nations (Rendall et al. 2005).

The figures in Table 2.1 are indicative only, due to differences in the way teenage pregnancies are calculated; the data for England and Wales and Scotland are for conceptions under 18, whereas the other countries present data for 15–19 year-olds. In addition, the latest data available for Canada are for 2011, not 2013.

The other issue to note when considering an overall figure for a country is that it hides the existence of large variability between different populations within some countries. Class is one indicator, as we have already seen, with working-class women having higher teenage birth rates than middle-class women, a pattern which holds true for all the countries being discussed, not just the UK. For 'New World' countries, race and ethnicity also play a role. For example, amongst First Nations women in Canada, 9 per cent of 15–19 year-olds are parents compared to 1.3 per cent of non-aboriginal Canadians (Eni and Phillips-Beck 2013). In the USA, the birth rate for 15–19 year-old African American women was 39 per 1000 women in 2013, compared to 18.6 per 1000 for White Americans (Department of Health and Human Services, Office of Adolescent Health 2015), while in Australia, the birth rate for Aboriginal 15–19 year-olds was 62.7 per 1000 compared to the national rate of 14.6 per 1000 (Australian Bureau of Statistics 2014). In New Zealand, Maori women under 25 have a birth rate double that of the whole population rate, but for women over 30 the Maori birth rate is much lower than the national rate (Families Commission 2012), suggesting that, like First Nations people in Canada, Maori people tend to start and complete their families earlier. The common factors linking the groups with birth rates above the relevant national figures, whether class or race, include educational attainment and employment status. First Nations, Maori and Aboriginal people are much less likely to complete post-compulsory education than their non-aboriginal counterparts, and find it much harder to obtain secure well-paid jobs. A study comparing Canada, Sweden, France, the UK and the USA (Singh et al. 2001) found that teenage pregnancy was associated with low income and low levels of education in all the countries studied, and a comparison of Britain and France found that the longer women stayed in education, not just the level of qualification obtained,

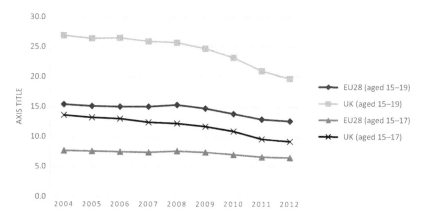

Fig. 2.2 Live birth rate (per 1000) to women in United Kingdom and EU28, 2004–2012. *Source*: ONS 2014b

influenced the shift towards the increase in the age at which women were having their first child (Ní Bhrolcháin and Beaujouan 2012). Countries with the greatest degree of income inequality experience the highest teenage pregnancy rates (UNICEF 2001).

The most recent comparative data for Europe (ONS 2014b) show that the birth rate for women aged 15–19 in the UK was 19.7 births per 1000 women in 2012, compared to a rate of 12.6 per 1000 for the EU28.[1] However, the UK birth rate (amongst teenagers) has been declining faster than birth rates elsewhere in Europe, with a 26.8 per cent fall since 2004, compared to 18.2 per cent for the EU28. Figure 2.2 illustrates the trends, showing a comparatively steep fall for births to 15–17 year-olds in the UK between 2008 and 2012.

As Table 2.1 shows, the most recent data for the USA indicate that in 2013, the birth rate for 15–19 year olds was 26.5 per 1000, a significant reduction from the figure in the UNICEF report but still the highest in the world (Department of Health and Human Services, Office of Adolescent Health 2015). The reductions in rates of teenage pregnancy

---

[1] The 'EU28' are the 28 nations comprising the European Union, which includes most of Western Europe (apart from Norway and Switzerland) and much of Eastern Europe apart from most of the Balkans.

over the last 15 years have been largest in those countries which had the highest rates in 1998, although they are still a long way from the countries which had the lowest rates. If the suggestion in the UNICEF report is correct, that less inclusive societies with higher degrees of income inequality have higher teenage pregnancy rates than more inclusive societies, then it may be difficult for countries such as the USA and the UK to maintain such falls in the current economic climate. In the UK in particular, the austerity agenda of the Coalition government is likely to be followed even more harshly by the Conservative government elected in May 2015, and inequalities seem to be widening rather than narrowing (Dorling 2015).

The Coalition Approach

The general election in the UK in 2010 resulted in a change of government, which occurred at what had been identified as the end point of the strategy, but obviously before any data for the whole period of its existence was available. The incoming Coalition government chose not to continue with a further strategy specifically for teenage pregnancy and parenting, but included the under-18 conception rate as one of the indicators in the *Public Health Outcomes Framework* (Department of Health 2013), and included the reduction of both under-18 and under-16 conception rates as a priority in the *Framework for Sexual Health Improvement* in England.

Upon election, the government embarked on wide-ranging reforms of the welfare system, including a proposal, subsequently enacted, to introduce a 'benefit cap'. This limited the amount of welfare benefits a family could claim, with the stated intention of ensuring that a family on benefits could never be better off than a typical family in work. This culminated in the Welfare Reform Act 2012 and associated regulations regarding different types of benefits and entitlements. The intention of the cap was to provide an incentive for people to find work, and to move if their housing costs were too high.

As well as introducing wide-reaching welfare reforms, the government also introduced the Troubled Families programme (DCLG 2012a, 2012b) in response to the riots in some UK cities in summer 2011. Crossley (2015) outlines how the concept of 'troubled families' is a natural successor to the ideas of families perpetuating cycles of deprivation, and underclass theories. Although the policy focus was on 'family', the emphasis fell on mothers, and in particular lone mothers who did not discipline their children, especially their sons, who were said to lack appropriate male role models. Prime Minister David Cameron connected single mothers and geographical localities in a speech after the riots when he said 'perhaps they come from one of the neighbourhoods where it's standard for children to have a mum and not a dad', (Cameron 2011) implicitly linking poor parenting with deprived neighbourhoods but placing the blame firmly on the shoulders of mothers.

Although the Troubled Families programme is consistent with long-standing state desires to deal with problem families, it differs from previous policy approaches in that it is not specific about age or marital status of mothers. Lone mothers are implicated as the sources of many of their family's problems (or, if not the source of the problem, the cause in their failure to tackle the problem, whether that is one of poor school attendance or criminal behaviour by their children), but the emphasis is on 'fixing' the family as a whole. Teenage parents, if they are mentioned at all, are mentioned as one of the symptoms of a troubled family.

Where Next with a Conservative Government in Power?

In May 2015, after a general election in the UK, the Coalition government was replaced by a Conservative government. Although there have been no announcements to date (July 2015) specifically about teenage pregnancy or parenting, it is likely that a continuation of the austerity agenda, with significant cuts planned to public spending including a lowering of the benefit cap and cuts to the public health budgets of local authorities, will impact not only on the benefits system but also on the services that help young people, both in terms of enabling access to contraceptive services, and supporting them if they become young parents. Family policy remains centred on the Troubled Families programme, which will be extended to cover more families.

During the course of the Coalition government, a number of Conservative MPs expressed views about teenage parents which hark back to the morality of previous decades; for example, the '40 Group', a group of 40 Conservative MPs in the 40 most marginal constituencies, produced a set of 40 policy ideas (Morris and Mowat 2013) including the suggestion that 'all benefits to teenage mothers should be made on the condition of them living with their parents or in supervised hostel accommodation' (2013, p. 75). This, they claimed, would stop teenagers deliberately becoming pregnant in order to be given a council house despite there being no evidence that this happens; they also ignore or are unaware of the fact that many teenage parents continue to live with their parents once their baby is born. The idea of mother and baby hostels is reminiscent of the mother and baby homes of the 1950s and 1960s discussed above, and in effect would mean that teenagers were denied the chance to establish themselves as a family, which somewhat undermines the Conservative party positioning itself as the party of the family. The danger of basing policies on particular views of morality was demonstrated by a previous Conservative government of 1992–1997, when Prime Minister John Major's much heralded (and subsequently derided) 'Back to Basics' approach was undermined by the sexual indiscretions of a number of Conservative MPs (BBC News 1998). Arai suggests that the Back to Basics campaign positioned young single mothers 'as the enemies of decent society' (2009, p. 57), and this Conservative view would not seem to have changed despite the efforts of party leader David Cameron to 'detoxify' the party, when he himself made speeches suggesting, as noted above, that the riots in some UK cities in summer 2011 were due to single mothers who do not monitor their children adequately.

Conclusions

The twentieth century saw massive shifts in attitudes towards motherhood and marriage, set in the broader social context of changes in women's lives, and changing attitudes towards sex and sexuality. Very few people in most Western democracies would now regard a child born outside marriage as being stained by illegitimacy, not least because in many countries, including England and Wales, increasing numbers of children are born outside marriage; in 2013, 47.4 per cent of births in England and Wales were outside marriage (ONS 2014a), and if current trends continue, by 2016 more births will be outwith than within marriage. Despite this, some aspects of motherhood remain contentious; there may have been a shift away from overt moralising about the right kind of mother, but commentary about who becomes a mother and at what age can often contain moralistic overtones. While young mothers are portrayed as being at fault for becoming a mother too young, older women are also criticised for leaving it too late, for selfishly putting themselves and their careers first, and then having to rely on IVF as well as being at a greater risk of complications for themselves and their baby. A steady stream of stories in the mainstream media appear to position motherhood as acceptable within a narrowing window of opportunity for a shrinking group of women.

What is striking from a review of attitudes to motherhood over more than a century, particularly problematic motherhood, is that on the one hand there have been radical shifts in outlook about issues such as pre-marital sex, illegitimacy and immorality, yet despite this some features of the debate reappear from time to time, albeit dressed in different clothes. We may no longer punish women who give birth outside marriage with banishment and incarceration in asylums (not least because the large Victorian asylums no longer exist), but media headlines, and politicians in need of hitting them with a sound bite, continue to demonise young mothers, single mothers, and the supposedly feckless men who father their babies. The other striking aspect of this review is how few mentions are made of men; the vast majority of policies and pronouncements focus on women. Assumptions that contemporary teenage parents will be unmarried are reasonable, given the decreasing popularity of marriage across the population as a whole, but assumptions that a teenage mother is automatically a lone mother, and that she is raising her baby without support, are inaccurate. Although most teenage parents are not married, most births to teenagers are registered by both parents; in 2010 40 per cent were joint registrations with parents living at the same address and 35 per cent were joint registrations with the parents living at different addresses (ONS 2011). Many also have support from their families, and are raising their child with the help of mothers, grandmothers, and other relatives.

One of the most significant changes has been around adoption; whereas in the first half of the twentieth century it was expected that a single mother (whatever her age) would give up her baby for adoption, this began to change in the 1960s, and now it is rare for a mother to give a newborn baby for adoption. This does not stop politicians suggesting that it would be preferable for both mother and baby if adoption became the norm once more, as John Redwood, former Conservative Welsh Secretary, argued in 1995, followed by Jack Straw, former Labour Home Secretary, saying in 1999 that babies would have a better life if their teenage mothers offered them for adoption. Most recently Martin Narey, Coalition government 'adoption tsar', suggested that it was wrong to tell pregnant teenagers that they would be able to cope with motherhood, and instead they should be encouraged to consider adoption.

The clearest move away from regarding teenage pregnancy and parenting as a moral issue, and its creation as a largely social problem, came with the then Labour government's Teenage Pregnancy Strategy of 1999. The strategy took an evidence-based approach, marshalling a considerable amount of data on the cause and outcomes of teenage pregnancy and parenting. However, this evidence is overwhelmingly quantitative and statistical; what is missing are the voices, the lived experiences, of teenage parents themselves. Graham and McDermott (2006) pointed out that quantitative evidence, which is most commonly used to inform policymaking, provides a largely negative view, but qualitative research with teenage parents, which provides a more nuanced and more positive outlook, is rarely called upon. The aim of this book is to provide such a qualitative perspective on teenage pregnancy and parenting from the people who have experience of it, and not only from the current generation of teenage parents, but also from those who have experienced the changing attitudes and views on teenage parenting over the decades by virtue of having been teenage parents in earlier times themselves.

References

Arai, L. (2009). *Teenage pregnancy: The making and unmaking of a problem.* Bristol: Policy Press.

Australian Bureau of Statistics. (2014). Births Australia 2013. Retrieved September 30, 2015, from http://www.abs.gov.au/AUSSTATS/abs@.nsf/Lookup/3301.0Main+Features12013?OpenDocument

BBC Democracy Live. (2014). Compulsory sex education rejected by peers. Retrieved September 30, 2015, from http://www.bbc.co.uk/democracylive/house-of-lords-25934084

BBC News. (1998). UK politics: The major scandal sheet. Retrieved September 30, 2015, from http://news.bbc.co.uk/1/hi/uk_politics/202525.stm

Cameron, D. (2011). Retrieved September 30, 2015, from https://www.gov.uk/government/speeches/pms-speech-on-the-fightback-after-the-riots

Carabine, J. (2007). New Labour's teenage pregnancy policy. *Cultural Studies, 21*(6), 952–973.

Centres for Disease Control and Prevention (CDC). (2007). *Teen birth rate rises for first time in 15 years.* Press release: US Department of Health and Human Statistics. Retrieved from http://www.cdc.gov/nchs/pressroom/07newsreleases/teenbirth.htm

Chandola, T., Coleman, D. A., & Hiorns, R. W. (2002). Heterogeneous fertility patterns in the English-speaking world. Results from Australia, Canada, New Zealand and the United States. *Population Studies, 56*(2), 181–200.

Conrad, D. (2012). Deprivation-based inequalities in under-18 conception rates and the proportion of under-18 conceptions leading to abortion in England, 1998–2010. *Journal of Public Health, 34*(4), 609–614.

Crossley, S. (2015). Realizing the (troubled) family, crafting the neoliberal state. *Families, Relationships and Societies.* doi:10.1332/204674315X14326465757666.

Department for Communities and Local Government. (2012a). *Financial framework for the Troubled Families programme's payment-by-results scheme for local authorities.* London: DCLG.

Department for Communities and Local Government. (2012b). *Listening to troubled families: A report by Louise Casey CBE.* London: DCLG.

Department for Education (DfE). (2010). *The importance of teaching: The schools white paper 2010.* London: Stationery Office.

Department for Education and Skills (DfES). (2006a). *Teenage pregnancy next steps: Guidance for local authorities and primary care trusts on effective delivery of local strategies.* London: Stationery Office.

Department for Education and Skills (DfES). (2006b). *Teenage pregnancy: Accelerating the strategy to 2010.* London: Stationery Office.

Department of Health. (1992). *The health of the nation – A strategy for health in England.* London: Stationery Office.

Department of Health. (2013). *Public health outcomes framework.* London: Stationery Office.

Department of Health and Human Services, Office of Adolescent Health. (2015). *Trends in teen pregnancy and childbearing.* Retrieved September 30, 2015, from http://www.hhs.gov/ash/oah/adolescent-health-topics/reproductive-health/teen-pregnancy/trends.html

Dorling, D. (2015). *Injustice: Why social inequality still persists* (2nd ed.). Bristol: Policy Press.

Duncan, S. (2007). What's the problem with teenage parents? And what's the problem with policy? *Critical Social Policy, 27*(3), 307–334.

Duncan, S., Edwards, R., & Alexander, C. (Eds.). (2010). *Teenage parenthood: What's the problem?* London: Tuffnell Press.

Eni, R., & Phillips-Beck, W. (2013). Teenage pregnancy and parenthood perspectives of first nation women. *The International Indigenous Policy Journal, 4*(1). Retrieved September 30, 2015, from http://ir.lib.uwo.ca/iipj/vol4/iss1/3

Families Commission. (2012). *Teenage pregnancy and parenting: An overview.* Wellington: New Zealand Families Commission.

Fraser, A. M., Brockert, J. E., & Ward, R. H. (1995). Association of young maternal age with adverse reproductive outcomes. *New England Journal of Medicine, 332*, 1113–1117.

Furstenberg, F. (2007). *Destinies of the disadvantaged. The politics of teenage childbearing.* New York: Russell Sage Foundation.

Galavotti, C., & Green, D. (2006). England's national teenage pregnancy strategy. *The Lancet, 368*, 1846–1848.

Graham, H., & McDermott, E. (2006). Qualitative research and the evidence base of policy: Insights from studies of teenage mothers in the UK. *Journal of Social Policy, 35*(1), 21–37.

Hadfield, L., Rudoe, N. and Sanderson-mann, J. (2007). Motherhood, choice and the British media: Time to reflect. *Gender and Education, 19*(2), 255–263.

Hadley, A. (2014). Teenage pregnancy: Huge progress … but more to do. *Community Practitioner, 87*(6), 44–47.

Hansard HL Deb 08 July 1992 vol 538 cc1183-98.

Hansard HL Deb 28 January 2014 vol 750 cc1118-55.

Hoggart, L. (2012). 'I'm pregnant … what am I going to do?' An examination of value judgements and moral frameworks in teenage pregnancy decision making. *Health, Risk and Society, 14*(6), 533–549.

Information Services Division. (2015). *Teenage pregnancy: Year of conception ending 31 December 2013*. NHS Scotland. Retrieved from http://www.isdscotland.org/Health-Topics/Maternity-and-Births/Teenage-Pregnancy/

Jivraj, S., Nazzal, Z., Davies, P., & Selby, K. (2010). Obstetric outcome of teenage pregnancies from 2002 to 2008: The Sheffield experience. *Journal of Obstetrics and Gynaecology, 30*(3), 253–256.

Johnson, A. (2014). *Please, Mr Postman: A memoir*. London: Penguin.

Macvarish, J. (2010). The effect of 'risk-thinking' on the contemporary construction of teenage motherhood. *Health, Risk & Society, 12*(4), 313–322.

McKay, A., & Barrett, M. (2010). Trends in teenage pregnancy rates from 1996 to 2006: A comparison of Canada, Sweden, USA and England/Wales. *Canadian Journal of Human Sexuality, 19*, 43–52.

Morris, J., & Mowat, D. (2013). *40 policy ideas from the 40*. London: Conservative Party.

Ní Bhrolcháin, M., & Beaujouan, E. (2012). Fertility postponement is largely due to rising educational enrolment. *Population Studies: A Journal of Demography, 66*(3), 311–327.

O'Hara, M. (2009). Teenage pregnancy rates rise. *The Guardian*. Retrieved September 30, 2015, from http://www.theguardian.com/society/2009/feb/26/teenage-pregnancy-rise

Office for National Statistics (ONS). (1998). *Population trends 93*. London: Stationery Office.

Office for National Statistics. (2006). *Population trends 126*. London: Stationery Office.

Office for National Statistics. (2011). *Frequently asked questions: Births and fertility, August 2011*. London: Stationery Office.

Office for National Statistics. (2014a). *Statistical bulletin: Births in England and Wales 2013*. London: Stationery Office.

Office for National Statistics. (2014b). *International comparisons of teenage pregnancy*. London: Stationery Office.

Office for National Statistics. (2015). *Statistical bulletin: Births in England and Wales 2014*. London: Stationery Office.

Olausson, P. O., Cnattingius, S., & Haglund, B. (1999). Teenage pregnancies and risk of late fetal death and infant mortality. *British Journal of Obstetrics and Gynaecology, 106*, 116–121.

Rendall, M., Couet, C., Lappegard, T., Robert-Bobée, I., Rønsen, M., & Smallwood, S. (2005). *Population trends: First births by age and education in Britain, France and Norway*. London: Office for National Statistics.

Singh, S., Darroch, J. E., & Frost, J. J. (2001). Socioeconomic disadvantage and adolescent women's sexual and reproductive behavior: The case of five developed countries. *Family Planning Perspectives, 33*(6), 251–258.

Sixsmith, M. (2009). *The lost child of Philomena Lee*. London: Macmillan.

Smith, G., & Pell, J. (2001). Teenage pregnancy and risk of adverse perinatal outcomes associated with first and second births: Population based retrospective cohort study. *British Medical Journal, 323*, 476–479.

Social Exclusion Unit (SEU). (1999). *Teenage pregnancy*. London: Stationery Office.

Social Exclusion Unit (SEU). (2004). *Breaking the cycle; taking stock of progress and priorities for the future*. London: Office of the Deputy Prime Minister.

Statistics Canada. (2013a). *Table 102-4503 – Live births, by age of mother, Canada, provinces and territories, annual*, CANSIM (database). Retrieved September 30, 2015, from http://www5.statcan.gc.ca/cansim/a34?lang=eng &mode=tableSummary&id=1024503&stByVal=2&p1=-1&p2=9

Statistics Canada. (2013b). *Table 102-4505 – Crude birth rate, age-specific and total fertility rates (live births), Canada, provinces and territories, annual (rate)*, CANSIM (database). Retrieved September 30, 2015, from http://www5. statcan.gc.ca/cansim/a26?lang=eng&retrLang=eng&id=1024505&tabMode =dataTable&srchLan=-1&p1=-1&p2=9

Statistics New Zealand. (2014). Births and deaths: Year ended December 2013. Retrieved September 30, 2015, from http://www.stats.govt.nz/browse_for_ stats/population/births/BirthsAndDeaths_HOTPYeDec13.aspx

Teenage Pregnancy Independent Advisory Group (TPIAG). (2010). *Teenage pregnancy: Past successes – Future challenges*. London: Department for Education.

Thane, P., & Evans, T. (2012). *Sinners? Scroungers? Saints? Unmarried motherhood in twentieth century England*. Oxford: Oxford University Press.

UNICEF. (2001). *A league table of teenage births in rich nations*. Innocenti Report Card No. 3. Florence: Innocenti Research Centre.

United Nations. (2003). *World fertility report*. Geneva: United Nations Department of Economic and Social Affairs, Population Division.

Universities of Leeds and Glamorgan and the London School of Hygiene and Tropical Medicine. (1998). *The Health of the Nation – A policy assessed*. London: Stationery Office.

Wellings, K., Wilkinson, P., Grundy, C., Kane, R., Lachowycz, K., Jacklin, P., et al. (2005). *Teenage pregnancy strategy evaluation final report synthesis*. London: Teenage Pregnancy Strategy Unit.

Whitley, R., & Kirmayer, L. J. (2008). Perceived stigmatisation of young mothers: An exploratory study of psychological and social experience. *Social Science and Medicine, 66*, 339–348.

Wilkinson, P., French, R., Kane, R., Lachowycz, K., Stephenson, J., Grundy, C., et al. (2006). Teenage conceptions, abortions, and births in England, 1994–2003, and the national teenage pregnancy strategy. *The Lancet, 368*, 1879–1886.

Wilson, H., & Huntington, A. (2006). Deviant (M)others: The construction of teenage motherhood in contemporary discourse. *Journal of Social Policy, 35*(1), 59–76.

3

'It Feels Like It's a Cultural Thing in This Area': The Study in Context

The research study that is discussed in the rest of this book explored the experiences of teenage parents across the generations, and decision-making about young parenthood, in families where grandparents and great-grandparents have themselves been teenage parents. The study was qualitative, and used a combination of in-depth focussed interviews and focus groups. I carried out fieldwork comprising interviews (individual, with seven young mothers and one older mother; and paired, with four mother and daughter pairs and one young mother and young father couple), four focus groups (with young parents and parents-to-be, and staff working with young people, and one family), and a limited amount of observation during 2012 and early 2013 in an industrial city in the north of England which was the main fieldwork site for the study. I held further focus groups with young people and with staff members in two other northern English cities and one city in the south-west, one focus group and an interview with staff in a city in Scotland, and three interviews (two staff members, one young mum) in South Wales. In this chapter, I describe the background to the study and how it was carried out, to enable the reader to understand the context of the research. As well as a brief discussion of the methods, the chapter will describe the settings

© The Editor(s) (if applicable) and The Author(s) 2016

S. Brown, *Teenage Pregnancy, Parenting and Intergenerational Relations*,
DOI 10.1057/978-1-137-49539-6_3

where the fieldwork took place, to provide geographical, social, economic and cultural contexts for the findings. I will also outline the theoretical perspectives that informed the research. As is conventional, in order to ensure anonymity, all the names of individuals taking part in the study have been changed, as have some minor details which do not affect the veracity of the research.

Inspiration

Prior to starting the work for this multigenerational study, I had carried out studies with young people where I talked to them about their use of contraception, attitudes towards contraception and risk taking, and feeling about issues such as sex education and abortion. As is often the case with focussed interviewing, indeed as is often desirable, some young people told stories about themselves and their lives that strayed from my semi-structured interview schedule. The first study (Brown and Guthrie 2010), which asked young women aged between 16 and 20 years old about their use of contraception, directly inspired a follow-up study with young men, as many of the young women started their remarks with phrases such as 'well, of course, all the boys say ...' and 'lads always ...' when talking about whose job it was to take responsibility for contraception. Many young women talked about the assumptions that they thought young men had, that the women would be on the pill, as well as young men's dislike of condoms. Having been told several times what 'all the boys say ...', my second study (Brown 2012) tried to find out what boys actually said. Did they say, or think, the things that the young women said they did? The story was, of course, rather more complex than that; decisions about responsibility for and use of contraception were nuanced, and often more to do with relationship status than with gender (Brown 2015a).

The inspiration for talking to people in families where more than one generation had experienced teenage pregnancy came directly from Lydia, a young woman in the first study. She was 17 years old and was having a termination of her second pregnancy, having had a baby when she was 15. She said:

My nana had my mam when she was 15, my mam had my brother when she was 15, and I had Jayden when I was 15. So it kind of like runs in the family.

So, of course, I wondered whether it does run in families, and if so, how do the families themselves work? What sort of decisions do they make, and how do they support their teenager, if indeed they do? Lydia went on to say that her mother, aged 34, had had a baby not long before Jayden was born, so she cared for both the young children to enable Lydia to return to college. Another young woman in the same study, interviewed at the age of 18 and with a baby born when she was 15, said:

Everyone knew, in my family, and they were all really excited, and wanted me to have the baby. So I did. And I know I shouldn't say I regret it, with her out there, but I do.

Natasha expressed regret now that she saw her friends going off to university and going on holidays, while she was working part-time in a shop, and living at home with her parents, her baby and her sisters, but her baby had been a wanted and welcomed baby, by her family at least. She decided to have a termination of her second pregnancy without telling anyone about it, to avoid any pressure from her family.

In the study with young men, none of whom were fathers, Sam, aged 17, suggested that cultures within families might influence the age at which people had children:

If your mam had you when she was young, you'd say 'well, it didn't do me any harm', so they get brought up to think it's OK to have a kid really young, and to think about having a kid when you're 30 is like another world. So I think it's the education you get as part of your upbringing.

Rob, who was 18 and, like Sam, at sixth form college, talked about not wanting to start a family until he had finished his education and got a job. Contrary to Sam's suggestion that growing up as the child of a teenage parent might be an encouragement to have children young, Rob explained that 'my mum was 18 when she had my older brother. But she said to me "don't do it"'.

There is a strong strand of thought, mainly from the political right, that sees the culture of families like Lydia's as faulty, and as perpetuating cycles of disadvantage, for example the writing of Charles Murray about the underclass, through Sir Keith Joseph's speeches in the 1970s and 1980s, to recent and ongoing newspaper headlines about 'benefit broods', automatically linking people who have several children with the benefits system and consequently with stigmatising and damaging labels. Missing from much of the political and media debate are the voices and lived experiences of the families, like Lydia's and Natasha's, and particularly the voices of young people, those like Sam and Rob without children, and those who we will hear from shortly who have them. The main aim of the research that forms this book was to explore how families with multigenerational experiences of teenage parenting talk about parenting, both becoming parents themselves and later, advising their children as they grow up. The second aim was to explore whether there is a culture around early parenting, and whether in some places it is actually encouraged, as some in the media would have us believe, or whether it is 'just something that happens round here'. As discussed in the previous chapter, the social exclusion agenda of the Labour Government of 1997–2010 had a geographical element to it, in that it identified that 'people *or areas*' (my emphasis) could experience a combination of different aspects of disadvantage such as high crime and poor housing. In addition, local authorities with the highest teenage pregnancy rates were identified as 'hotspots', again a geographical identification of a place that had a problem that needed to be solved. The research, therefore, began in one such hotspot, and then other sites and settings were added due to them being 'statistical neighbours' in England of the original city, as well as places that had been identified as hotspots in Scotland and Wales. Statistical neighbours are local authorities who have similar outcomes for a particular indicator; the concept was originally developed to help local authorities in carrying out benchmarking and comparative studies. For teenage pregnancy, each local authority will have five statistical neighbours who are their closest statistically at that point in time in terms of rates for pregnancies under 18; obviously these neighbours can change, depending on how individual local authorities' pregnancy rates change, so over a period of years, a local authority is likely to be neighbour to more than five others. These neighbours are often not geographically close, although as teenage pregnancy rates are higher in urban deprived areas in the north, and in London, London boroughs tend to have other London boroughs as neighbours, and northern towns mainly have other northern towns. For example, Lambeth, which in 1999 had the highest teenage pregnancy rate in the country, has statistical neighbours who are also geographically close: Southwark, Hackney, Lewisham, Haringey and Newham. Middlesbrough, which has in several years been amongst the ten local authorities with the highest teenage pregnancy rates, has Hartlepool, Stockton-on-Tees, Sunderland, Redcar and Cleveland, and South Tyneside as statistical neighbours, all of whom who are in the same region. In contrast, Liverpool's statistical neighbours include Hull, Belfast, Salford and Plymouth.

The Settings

In order to maintain confidentiality, especially as in some places only a few people took part in interviews and focus groups, the names of the locations have been changed, and most of the data I have used is nationally available data from sources such as the ONS, and the Welsh and Scottish Governments' statistics agencies. Where data has originated from the local authorities themselves, the references have not been included in the bibliography in order to allow the locations to remain anonymised. What follows is a description of the places in the study, and a discussion of their similarities and differences. It should be noted that the purpose of providing data about the locations is not in order to do a comparative data analysis, but to establish a picture of the places and the challenges they face, in terms of indicators of multiple deprivation and some of the factors included in the SEU's definition of social exclusion, particularly levels of educational attainment and unemployment. In addition, it should also be noted that the data provided can sometimes mask the wide variations within and across the locations that are known to the people who work there; for example, staff in several locations could identify small areas within their cities that had particularly high rates of teenage pregnancy compared to other areas.

Seaborough, Milton and Norland are all in the north of England, Seaborough on the north-east coast, Milton and Norland in the north-west. Barton, on the south coast, has a number of similarities with Seaborough and with Bridgetown in Scotland in that all three have a maritime history, with trawler fishing, shipping and shipbuilding, and the Royal and Merchant Navy having been major employers in the past. Milton, like Carville in Wales, has had an industrial past, both being locations for heavy industries which have now more or less ceased to exist. All had been identified at some point during the history of the TPS as being amongst the local authorities having the highest teenage pregnancy rates in the UK, and all had had the infrastructure of the strategy in place until 2010, although by 2012 restructuring, cuts and reorganisations within local authorities had begun to take their toll, with reductions in staff numbers and changes in staff roles.

As Fig. 3.1 shows, all the locations had conception rates amongst under 18-year-olds above the national rate in 1999, when the strategy began, and these were still above the national figure in 2013; however, all areas showed a significant decrease, and all were much closer to the national figure than they had been previously. The 'blip' in the national rate in 2007, which caused the flurry of media stories mentioned in Chapter 2,

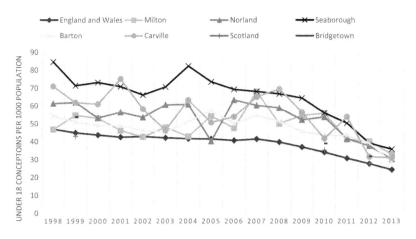

Fig. 3.1 Conception rates for under 18-year-olds per 1000 population, 1998–2013. *Source*: ONS (2014a), ISD (2015)

also shows up in the rates for Milton and Barton, but not in Seaborough or Norland, where the downward trend continued, and not in Carville, where the peak of the blip occurred a year later, before rates resumed their downward trend. Figure 3.1 also demonstrates one of the hazards of dealing with relatively small numbers, in that fluctuations between years can look like a very dramatic change in rates. The important point to note is that despite fluctuations, which in the case of Carville with a relatively small population compared to the English locations seem very dramatic as depicted in Fig. 3.1, all areas had a significant fall in rates and, overall, had established a downward trend over the period of the strategy's existence, and this has continued to date.

The fact that the local authorities were all reliant on heavy industry, manufacturing and shipping for a significant proportion of jobs in their areas meant that they had all been badly affected by the recession in 2008, and in some cases had barely begun to recover from previous downturns. It is well established that for large parts of the north of England, Scotland and South Wales, where 'deindustrialisation is a fundamental driver of poor health' (Taulbut et al. 2011), long-term decline has resulted in high rates of unemployment and incapacity across generations. Areas that were hardest hit by previous deindustrialisation were particularly badly affected by economic conditions between 2008 and 2010 (Elliott et al. 2010) and recovery from recession was predicted to be, and has been, unequal (Audit Commission 2009), with the resulting consequences for unemployment rates. In 2012, when most of the fieldwork took place, the unemployment rate for the UK as a whole was 7.9 per cent, slightly higher for Scotland at 8 per cent and Wales at 8.4 per cent. All the study locations had higher rates, with only Barton coming close to the national average, as Table 3.1 shows.

Rates of economic inactivity, an indicator of those who are not working and not looking for work, often due to long-term illness, or to being a carer or an at-home parent, were also higher than the national average in all locations apart from Barton.

Young people were particularly badly affected during the recession which began in 2008, in terms of youth unemployment being higher than the 'all age groups' headline figure used in the table. Table 3.1 shows the percentage of 18–24 year-olds claiming Jobseeker's Allowance (JSA), and

Table 3.1 Unemployment rates and JSA claimant rates, 2012

	Unemployment rate 2012 (%)	JSA claimants 18–24 year olds (%)
Great Britain	7.9	7.3
Scotland	8	8.2
Wales	8.4	8
Seaborough	15.4	13.8
Barton	8.2	6.5
Milton	10.9	12.1
Norland	9.6	9.1
Carville	12.1	14.2
Bridgetown	10.1	9.0

Source: ONS (2013) and NOMIS (2015)

in all the study areas, it was higher than the national average in 2012. The JSA claimant figure is likely to be lower than the actual number of young people being unemployed, as those who are unemployed but not claiming, for whatever reason, do not appear in these statistics. As we will hear in Chapter 7, the complexities of the types of employment available in the locations and to the young people there, along with the benefits system, were felt to be challenging for young parents to negotiate. One of the key indicators of how well an area can recover from recession is the rate of applicants per job; where this is high, it suggests that not enough jobs are being created for the available workforce. It also may lead to disillusionment amongst applicants, particularly those who have few educational qualifications, which again may impact particularly heavily on young people in the study areas. Seaborough had one of the highest applicants per job ratio in the UK in 2010, combined with lower than average attainment rates at GCSE. The local authority felt that this suggested a mismatch between people and jobs, with people looking for low-skilled work that was no longer available, and not having the qualifications needed to obtain more skilled work. One consequence, suggested by one of the staff members there, was that young people might decide to 'sit out' the recession, and have children while there were no jobs available to them, in the hope that the economy would pick up and they would get a job later. However, none of the young people described their situation this way, and we will hear more about how they viewed their trajectories through work, education and parenthood later.

Indices of multiple deprivation data (DCLG 2011) indicate that in 2010 Seaborough had over 40 per cent of its Lower Layer Super Output Areas (LSOAs)[1] in the most deprived 10 per cent while Norland had a third; both Carville and Bridgetown had high rates of deprivation relative to Wales and Scotland respectively. Given that income, employment and education are key domains in determining the indicators, it is unsurprising that the local authorities in the study contain some of the most deprived areas. It is also predictable, given the connections made by the SEU in 1999 between social deprivation and teenage pregnancy, that the study locations are those with some of the highest rates across the UK at various points during the lifetime of the strategy.

The links between education, unemployment and teenage pregnancy are well established, but as discussed in Chapter 2, the mechanisms are less clear, with views about the existence of causation, never mind the direction, being contentious. While it seems obvious that having schooling interrupted by pregnancy will have implications for future employability, this may be less significant for young women who had neither plans nor desire to remain in education. While some may be incentivised by the lack of good jobs to work harder, in order to improve their chances of getting one of the few available, others may feel that there is little point in pursuing qualifications for jobs that simply do not exist in their area.

Poor skills and low incomes were two of the factors in the SEU's description of the components of social exclusion, and Table 3.2 shows the percentages of people (aged 16–64) with no qualifications and those with NVQ2 and above (that is, those who have five or more GCSEs at grades A–C or the equivalent), along with the average weekly earnings per employed adult, in each of the study locations.

All the study locations apart from Barton have higher percentages of people with no qualifications, and lower percentages of those with the equivalent of five GCSEs at grades A–C, which is a widely accepted standard of a minimum educational qualification, than the national average. Those who have not attained that standard will find anything other than

---

[1] LSOAs are geographic areas designed to make reporting of small area statistics in local authorities in England and Wales more accurate. Each LSOA has a population of between 1000 and 3000 people. They replace statistics being reported at electoral ward level as wards varied greatly in size so were not easily comparable.

Table 3.2 Qualifications and earnings, 2012

	No qualifications (%)	NVQ2 and above (%)	Weekly earnings per adult (£)
Great Britain	9.7	71.8	508
Scotland	9.4	73.1	498
Wales	11.4	69.7	455
Seaborough	16.2	63.6	432
Barton	6.2	72.5	452
Milton	12.1	65.8	418
Norland	12.1	67.5	454
Carville	14.6	62.4	412
Bridgetown	13	68.5	432

Source: NOMIS (2015)

low-skilled work hard to obtain. Unsurprisingly, as the locations have a population with lower skills, the average weekly earnings are also lower. Barton stands out, though, as a local authority with slightly above average levels of education, yet with a low average weekly wage. The important point to note is that this figure is the average for all adults in full-time employment; young people are likely to earn less than this, and women and people who work part-time are likely to have a lower average hourly rate of pay; this suggests that young parents who can work are likely to be earning much less than the figures given above.

Poor health is another of the SEU's indicators of social exclusion, and Table 3.3 shows life expectancy (LE) and disability-free life expectancy (DFLE) at birth and at age 65, and the percentage of people whose day-to-day activities are limited by ill health.

Although these are very broad statistics which do not show any in-area variations, which can be considerable as we know from examples such as the 'Glasgow effect' (Walsh et al. 2010), they still paint a picture of the study locations having a shorter life expectancy at birth and at age 65 than for the national averages; they also show that people can expect to live less healthy lives as well as shorter ones. For example, a 65-year-old woman in Wales can expect to live for another 20 years, but only just over half of those years will be disability-free. A baby girl born in Seaborough in the period covered by the table might expect to live until the age of 80, but her healthy life expectancy is just 57 years. Further demonstration

Table 3.3 Life expectancy, disability-free life expectancy, and limitation of daily activities, 2011–2013

	LE at birth (m)	LE at birth (f)	DFLE at birth (m)	DFLE at birth (f)	LE at 65 (m)	LE at 65 (f)	DFLE at 65 (m)	DFLE at 65 (f)	Daily activities limited (% of population)
England	79.4	83.1	63.3	63.9	18.56	21.1	10.9	12.2	17.6
Scotland	75.8	80	59.3	64.5	16.6	19.2	9	11.1	19.7
Wales	78.2	82.2	63.5	65.3	18	20	10	11	22.7
Seaborough	76.6	80.7	57.4	56.9	16.5	19.4	7.5	8.2	19.6
Barton	78.2	82.4	58.3	59.4	17.8	20.6	8.4	10.3	20.4
Milton	77.3	80.4	58.3	61	16.7	19.5	8.6	9.9	21.4
Norland	76.6	80.4	57.9	58.8	16.2	19.1	7.5	8.4	20.7
Carville	76.9	80.9	57.9	59.6	17	19.6	b	b	27
Bridgetown[a]	71.6	78	64.6	68.6	14.7	18	11.5	13.7	21

Source: ONS (2014), Stats Wales (2013), ISD (2014)
[a]Data based on 2001 census
[b]Data not available below All Wales level

that people in the study locations live not only shorter lives but lives with more disability and illness is provided by the final column, which shows the percentage of the population whose daily activities are limited by ill health: 17.6 per cent for England, compared to 20 per cent or more for most of the study areas, rising to 27 per cent for Carville.

In her paper examining how teenage parenting relates to culture and identity, in particular amongst urban African Americans, Geronimus suggests that early childbearing may be an adaptive strategy for a population facing a shorter healthy life expectancy than the norm (Geronimus 2003). The mothers in Burton's (1990) study, also in the USA, perceived themselves to have a shorter than average life expectancy, therefore could see no reason to postpone childbearing. Indeed, they may have felt an imperative to start a family early. If the shorter life expectancy experienced in the locations for my study influences patterns of childbearing, we would expect to see more women giving birth than the national average at a young age, and fewer than the average in the older age groups, and this appears to be true. Comparing patterns of childbearing nationally and regionally for England and Wales shows some differences which may relate to family structure in terms of when having a family begins and ends, as Fig. 3.2 shows.

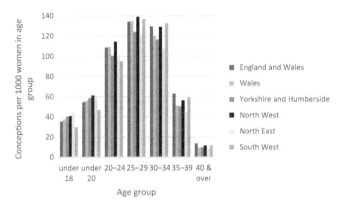

Fig. 3.2 Age of mother and area of residence, 2012. *Source*: ONS (2012)

Although each individual area has a similar shaped bell curve, the patterns at the extremes are interesting. The first column in each grouping shows the birth rate for England and Wales for that age group. For under-18, under- 20, and 20–24 age groups, the rate for England and Wales is below the rates for Wales, the North East, the North West, and Yorkshire and Humberside; in other words, the birth rate in those regions for those age groups is above the national average. At the other end of the chart, the birth rate for those regions has dropped below average by the age of 30, and for all age groups above 30 remains below the national average. The overall birth rates for Wales (73.8 per 1000 women aged 15–44), Yorkshire and Humberside (75.6) and the North East (71.7) were below the England and Wales rate of 78.5 per 1000 women, with the North West slightly above at 79.6. This suggests that women in these regions, which contain many of the hotspots for teenage pregnancy, are starting and completing their families earlier than the national average, but not that they have more children. In contrast, the South West reflects the national pattern, with below average rates of birth for younger women, and higher rates for older women. This suggests that Barton, as a hotspot, is an anomaly within the South West, which may account for its statistical neighbours being in the north rather than being geographically close. Unfortunately, figures are not available down to local authority level, but it seems reasonable to surmise that, given that the local authorities that are study locations have high teenage pregnancy rates, they will reflect this start-early/finish-early pattern.

The Settings Summarised

The data above paints a picture where for most, if not all, of the key indicators used to define areas of the UK as experiencing social exclusion, the study areas score poorly. They have higher rates of unemployment than the national average, their populations have fewer qualifications and more of them have no qualifications at all. As a consequence, many of them earn significantly below the national average wage. Much of this is due to the consequences of the recession which began in 2008, with many of the locations still struggling at that point to recover from previous downturns. All the locations have a shorter life expectancy for their populations, and people there expect to spend more of their life in poor health or with their daily activities limited by ill health. People tend to start their families earlier and complete them sooner than the national average, although they do not have larger families.

All this paints a very bleak and depressing picture, and would lead naturally to a belief that the quantitative approach to assessing the impact of teenage pregnancy and parenting provides an accurate representation of the hazards and detriments of early childbirth. However, as the following chapters will show, although there are difficulties and challenges in becoming a young parent, there is also joy and pleasure, and the depressing impression given by the bare numbers is rarely reflected in how people talk about their lives. Graham and McDermott (2006) made the point that qualitative findings are often overlooked in the policy world in favour of quantitative data; the purpose of the rest of this book is to add to the qualitative data and in so doing add insights and understanding about how people make decisions about parenthood, how they become parents and how families work in these settings. Before we move on to hear what they said, I will explain how the inspiration I discussed earlier became, in a practical sense, the study that forms the basis of this book.

Hearing People's Stories

Merely describing how fieldwork is conducted, and how 'data' are gathered, has been insufficient in sociology at least since Oakley discussed the methodological issues involved in interviewing women about motherhood, particularly the mismatch between the idea of an interviewer as data-gatherer, and a feminist-informed research practice which seeks to collect stories that validate women's experiences (Oakley 1981). More recently, again reflecting on research about motherhood, Thomson says 'we must remember that methodology shapes the kind of relationships that are evident, and that methods and theories are part of the context that produces what comes to be sociological "knowledge"' (Thomson 2009, p. 1). Thomson cites Back's assertion of the need for ethnographic methods involving 'the craft of engaged listening and descriptive writing' (Thomson 2009, p. 1) which can reflect 'the enigmatic and shifting nature of social existence' (Back 2007, p. 153) in order to produce a 'literary sociology that aims to document and understand social life, without assassinating it' (Back 2007, p. 164).

My methodology undoubtedly shaped the relationships between me as researcher and the people I was interviewing, and at times was a source of confusion for people who sought to understand what I was doing and why. One such example occurred when I visited a family one evening, and describing what happened also serves to illustrate how people came to be part of the study; how my participants were recruited, in the formal language of methodology sections. All my initial contacts were made via the Teenage Pregnancy Unit (TPU) in Seaborough; in late 2011 and early 2012, young women attending the service for the first time were asked if they knew how old their mother was when she had her first baby. If they said she had been in her teens, they were then asked if they would like to participate in the study, and if so, could their phone number be passed to me (usually described as 'a researcher from the university'). The first eight phone numbers resulted in three unanswered calls, one unreturned message, two people saying they had changed their minds, and two young women saying yes, I could go to see them. Further rounds of this style of recruitment, whereby the workers at the TPU acted as intermediaries for me, gradually resulted in all the participants we will hear from in this book agreeing that I could go to see them. It is worth noting that when I first approached the TPU, staff there were confident that they would be able to find plenty of respondents, as they were sure that many of the teenagers who used the service were themselves the children of teenage mothers. However, when it came to asking the teenagers themselves, they found that in fact, although many mothers had been young, in terms of the average age of mothers at first birth, they had not been teenagers; it was more common for mothers to have been in their early twenties. McNulty (2010) came up against the same issue in recruitment for her study; health professionals assumed that teenage parenting across three generations was much more common than it actually was.

Most people understood that I would be interviewing them, but did not really know why I was interested, and 'I don't know if I've told you the right answers' was not an unusual comment. This notion of the right answer was highlighted by my experience of interviewing one family; I arrived at their home in the early evening expecting to meet Debbie, a pregnant 17-year-old, and her mother, as arranged. On arrival, I found Debbie's grandmother Eileen and her great-aunt also waiting. 'You're here to do a survey', Eileen said. I explained that I was not doing a survey, I was doing some interviews with young mums. It then emerged that Debbie had thought I was going to be testing her on her knowledge of childcare, and had asked her grandmother to come round and ask hard questions about babies in order to prepare her for the test that I would be setting. As I reassured them that I would not be setting any tests, or giving any reports to anyone about whether or not Debbie was capable of being a good mum, I had to explain what I did actually want; 'I'm interested in family life,' I said. So everyone settled down around the dining table to talk about family life, and what had been planned as an interview turned into a family focus group. (I have explored this idea of 'naturally occurring focus groups' further elsewhere; see Brown 2015b). Sometimes researchers have to be quick on their feet, it seems, but for me, the serendipity of a whole family being there and being willing to talk to me about their lives, once I had explained what I was doing, was one of the benefits of taking an ethnographic, exploratory approach to understanding family life. As other qualitative researchers have found, the idea that researchers want an answer, rather than to understand the enigmatic nature of social life, as Back says, was common.

When I spoke to the teenagers, I asked if their mothers and/or partners would also be interested in taking part, and in several cases this resulted in joint interviews. I also asked if I could return four to six months later for a follow-up interview, and thus managed to see five people twice; one family agreed but could not be contacted later, and one family agreed but then did not respond to invitation letters. The second-round interviews introduced a temporal element to the research, and enabled the exploration of change in people's lives, in particular whether they had been able to do things they had said they wanted to, such as return to college or move house. It also seemed to introduce an element of growing trust; as discussed above, some people were uncertain about what I was doing and why, and this had led to some wariness on their part at first, or at least, I perceived them as being wary. The difference between the interviews also reflected Cornwell's findings about public and private accounts, whereby public accounts are often direct answers to direct questions, and private accounts happen when people are asked to tell a story, and focus more on the story than the audience (Cornwell 1984). The advantage of the second interview was that people gave more revealing replies, in terms of the stories they told and how they felt. No longer puzzled about my interest in family life, they knew I must be interested in what they had to say, and not 'right answers', because I had gone back to talk to them again.

Planned focus groups also took place at the TPU in Seaborough, one during a regular young parents' drop-in session, and one during an antenatal drop-in session. I attended the drop-in session the previous week, and talked informally about what I was doing, then returned the following week so that young people had had a week's warning in case they did not want to participate. Another serendipitous focus group occurred when the staff at the drop-in centre said 'you can interview us too', so I returned the following week to carry out another focus group during their lunch break. Both the planned and serendipitous focus groups took place in naturally occurring settings; the added benefit of taking the research to where people are, rather than expecting the participants to come to the researcher, is that people take part who might not otherwise feel able to, or simply could not have made the journey had the focus groups taken place at the university, for example.

The second part of the study aimed to explore whether there was a culture in some areas around teenage pregnancy; as outlined in Chapter 2, there is a view that in some areas, including the hotspots, teenage pregnancy is accepted, and possibly encouraged. One of the themes that had emerged during the fieldwork in Seaborough was a sense that 'it is something that happens round here', so with the help of one of the teenage pregnancy coordinators, I contacted coordinators in local authorities that were or had recently been statistical neighbours of Seaborough to see if they would be interested in taking part. Unfortunately this part of the study coincided with major upheavals across the health and welfare sectors, as Public Health Departments moved out of the NHS and into local authorities, people lost their jobs or changed roles as a result of the reorganisation, and responsibilities for teenage pregnancy services became fragmented. As a result, fieldwork could not take place in some local authorities simply because at the point I contacted them, no-one was actively responsible for a single joined-up service. However, in three locations in England, one in Scotland and one in Wales, people were able to help and expressed interest in taking part, so phase two included focus groups and interviews with staff and young people in the five locations described above. Again, the initial contact was with the staff, and they asked young people if they would be interested in talking to me, and if so, set up a meeting. At this point, not all the young people who took part were the child of a teenage parent, but the focus on this part of the study was on local cultures and experiences of current teenage parents in those places.

Although there was a certain amount of randomness in terms of the people who took part in the study, they were not randomly selected in a formal sense, and in that way my approach reflects that of Cornwell when she says that her cases:

> were not randomly selected and cannot therefore be regarded as 'typical' or 'representative' in the statistical sense. They are however 'typical' in the colloquial meaning of the word: their lives faithfully reflect the history of social and economic life in East London over the past eighty or more years. (Cornwell 1984, p. 1)

My study does not aim to be representative, nor am I making any claims for generalisability; by going to the statistical neighbours of Seaborough I was not attempting triangulation. The stories told here are, however, illustrative of a set of experiences around teenage pregnancy and parenting that may be transferable to other settings, and may illuminate similar cultures and experiences.

Analysis and Story-Building

All the interviews and focus groups were recorded, with the consent of the participants, and then transcribed. I also took fieldnotes at the focus groups, and made notes after the interviews and after some informal conversations. Everyone I spoke to in the locations knew I was doing research about teenage parents, and my identity as 'the girl from the university' (Richards and Emslie 2000) was undoubtedly helpful, even though some people found it puzzling that someone would want to talk about ordinary life. Analysis of the transcripts commenced by using a constant comparison approach (Strauss and Corbin 1990) to code and categorise data, and to identify themes emerging from the data. These themes structured the initial analysis, and also informed ongoing data generation, in that topics which were important to participants were pursued in later interviews and focus groups. For some key themes I then turned to a thematic narrative analysis approach (Riessman 1993, 2008), partly because as Prior (2011) found in his study with young people, participants' narratives took the form of stories about their experiences: things that had happened at the bus stop, comments they had overheard, and how they had responded or reacted. This 'story-building' aimed at having a story based on particular experiences to inform the writing up of the research, as well as stories of individuals and families. Storytelling was common across interviews and focus groups, and often about the same topics: stigma, judgemental people and being a good mother were mentioned frequently.

The differences between interviews and focus groups reflected the differing intensity of the situation; when I was talking to only one or two people in an interview, they told more personal stories, unsurprisingly, and with more detail about their life histories. Participants in focus groups talked about their own experiences, but also compared and contrasted themselves with each other, and with other people of their acquaintance, as well as telling stories about things they had seen on television, in the newspaper or on social media. This was most often done in positioning themselves as good mothers, when they used a 'bad people exist but I'm not one of them' discourse (Kingfisher 1996, p. 56). As the discussions later will show, young parents in the focus groups were engaged in identity work in ways that they were not when interviewed individually. This may reflect Wenham's finding, which I also found, that the young people were acutely aware of the social disapproval attached to the identity of teenage parent, and they were 'highly attuned to what people thought of them and why they might be treated differently from others.' (Wenham 2015, p. 9). The discourse and the identity work serve to both acknowledge and distance themselves from the stigma and social disapproval, and in the performative setting of a focus group they are working to present a particular image, even when they are surrounded by their peers.

Theoretical Frameworks

This study is situated within a constructionist perspective, a theoretical approach which seeks to explore what is happening in a social world (in this case the social world of young parents) by looking at how ordinary, everyday procedures and interactions produce social realities, and how people construct and manage their social worlds through both their practical activity and discourses (Holstein and Gubrium 2008; Silverman 2013). Narrative analysis enables the accounts given by participants to be seen as stories told about circumstances and events which took place in local contexts; the narrators (participants) place themselves in a story, and position themselves in relation to others (Riessman 2011). In this study the stories are about becoming and being a parent, the contexts are the immediate social settings as well as the towns or cities in which participants live, and the relational aspects are both the family relationships and how the young people relate to others in their social settings. The concept of capital, in social, cultural and economic forms (Bourdieu 1986) has also provided a way of analysing how individuals construct their worlds in their new role (as a parent) and in their relationships, both familial and in the context of wider society. Holland (2009) reviewed the uses of the concept of social capital in youth studies. She pointed out the problems with its adoption by a number of different academic disciplines as well as by policymakers, particularly where 'building and enhancing social capital has been seen as a magic bullet for difficult policy issues' (Holland 2009, p. 334) such as tackling social exclusion. She suggested that two broad camps exist in work on social capital and young people: those who use it as a concept 'dealing with the dilemma of collective action and integration' (2009, p. 333), and those who are interested in social justice and inequality, following Bourdieu. Placing herself in the second camp, she argued that social capital is a useful concept in 'encapsulating the types of processes and practices that are important for understanding the lives of young people, families and communities, and the connections between the micro and macro social' (2009, p. 345). As Scambler also points out, 'Bourdieu intended his work to be a means of exploring and seeking to explain empirical data' (Scambler 2012, p. 79), and for it to provide tools to think about how the world works. It is in this sense, as a useful set of tools to explore processes and practices in the lives of young parents, and the social contexts in which they operate, that I have used it in my analysis.

The study is informed by a number of bodies of work within sociology and social policy, including studies about and theoretical perspectives on family, youth transitions (particularly work on critical moments) and stigma. Daly and Kelly (2015) outline the shift in scholarship on the family away from a view of family as institution towards a focus on relationships and activities. The concept of family practices (Morgan 1996, 2013) looks at everyday interactions, and considers how these interact to create the meaning of family with fluid rather than fixed boundaries (Williams 2004). Here, family is about 'doing' rather than 'being' any particular set-up (such as the idealised nuclear family), and a family exists where people undertake activities together which they utilise in defining themselves as a family. Thus, a family could be an unmarried couple who live separately but raise a child together, 'doing' family in the way they attend parents' evenings or doctor's appointments together, for example. Chapter 6 explores the concept of family practices in more depth.

The concept of transitions has been described by MacDonald and colleagues as one which is 'hotly contested' (MacDonald et al. 2005, p. 874) within the sociology of youth studies. From the perspective of theories of individualism and the risk society (Beck 1992) which see transitions as fragmented and extended, structurally oriented and class-based approaches do not make sufficient allowance for individual autonomy or for the variations in paths to adulthood. However, MacDonald and colleagues argue that the concept remains a valuable one because young people's destinations in adulthood are still strongly influenced by their position in the class structure. In addition, they note the need to prioritise the accounts of young people about how they make decisions and create their transitions.

Two other concepts have informed how transitions occur for the young people in this study, firstly that of the critical moment and secondly, that of stigma. Rachel Thomson and colleagues developed the concept of a critical moment in a young person's process of transition to adulthood as an event that they could identify as having 'important consequences for their lives and identities' (2002, p. 339). In the context of the stories told by the young people in this study, the critical moments of pregnancy and the birth of a baby marked a transition from adolescence to adulthood, from being someone who had few, if any, responsibilities, to becoming someone with huge responsibility for a wholly dependent baby. These transitions and the critical moments of having to grow up are explored in depth in Chapter 8.

Since Goffman's (1963) initial work on stigma, a considerable body of work exploring theories of health-related stigma has developed, with the concepts having been explored and extended most notably by Graham Scambler. According to Scambler and colleagues (Scambler and Hopkins 1986; Scambler and Paoli 2008) there are three key dimensions to stigma: enacted stigma exists where one group is seen by another, more powerful group as imperfect or deviant; felt stigma is experienced by the 'imperfect' group in terms of an internalised sense of shame because they sense the perceptions held about them; project stigma is having a set of strategies as a form of resistance against enacted stigma. In addition, Scambler emphasised the need to account for the influence of social and structural factors, particularly the prejudices arising from the adoption of specific stereotypes by the general population, which he refers to as public stigma (Scambler 2004, 2009). The young parents and parents-to-be are well aware of the stigmatising discourses around teenage parenthood, dependency on the welfare state, and benefits claimants. As we will see in Chapter 4, they know from the point at which they become pregnant that their transition to adulthood is occurring within a framework of public and enacted stigma. The recurring themes of surveillance and being judged by those around them are woven through the stories told by the participants in this study.

A further theme recurs throughout the book, and that is the role of the welfare state, particularly the benefits system, in a context of austerity policies introduced by neoliberal governments. These concepts require definition for the purposes of clarity, not least because some, like neoliberalism, are sometimes used in a loose shorthand where the meaning is vague. The origins of neoliberalism may be found in the monetarist approach of Hayek and Friedman, an approach which gives primacy to markets and laissez-faire ideology, and challenges notions of a Keynesian welfare state. Those governments which could be said to be neoliberal, primarily the UK and the USA, favour, in theory at least, a minimal role for the state, in particular the reduction of state support for a broad range of welfare provision, while offering what Tyler refers to as the 'rhetoric of individualism, choice, freedom, mobility and national security' (2013, p. 7). Tyler's critique of how neoliberal governments work is instructive, in particular the way they operate to stigmatise and demonise certain groups; as this book will show, teenage parents are one such group. Austerity is used as a policy approach by neoliberal governments, ostensibly by cutting welfare spending in order to reduce budget deficits and support economic recovery following the worldwide recession of 2008. Some authors, of whom Tyler is one, would argue that austerity is in fact ideologically driven, with a view to reducing the role of the state to a 'nightwatchman' and removing welfare provision. This is done in part by reintroducing notions of 'deserving' and 'undeserving' poor, whereby those in receipt of state help are stigmatised as undeserving, which then provides a rationale for removing the support. For the purposes of this book, a neoliberal approach can be understood as one that favours markets and individualism over public welfare provision and collectivism, that is pursuing austerity as an ideological project, and that wishes to reduce the role of the welfare state while denigrating those who rely on it.

Having discussed teenage pregnancy and parenting in historical and policy contexts, and introduced the locations for the study, it is now time to hear from the young people themselves, their families, and the people who work with them.

References

Audit Commission. (2009). *When it comes to the crunch: How councils are responding to the recession*. London: Audit Commission.

Back, L. (2007). *The art of listening*. Oxford: Berg.

Beck, U. (1992). *Risk Society: Towards a new modernity*. London: Sage.

Bourdieu, P. (1986). The forms of capital. In J. Richardson (Ed.), *Handbook of theory and research for the sociology of education*. New York: Greenwood.

Brown, S. (2012). Young men, sexual health, and responsibility for contraception: A qualitative pilot study. *Journal of Family Planning and Reproductive Healthcare, 38*(1), 44–47.

Brown, S. (2015a). 'They think it's all up to the girls': Gender, risk and responsibility for contraception. *Culture, Health & Sexuality, 17*(3), 312–325.

Brown, S. (2015b). Using focus groups in naturally occurring settings. *Qualitative Research Journal, 15*(1), 86–97.

Brown, S., & Guthrie, K. (2010). Why don't teenagers use contraception? A qualitative interview study. *European Journal of Contraception and Reproductive Health Care, 15*, 197–204.

Burton, L. (1990). Teenage childbearing as an alternative life-course strategy in multigeneration black families. *Human Nature, 1*(2), 123–143.

Cornwell, J. (1984). *Hard earned lives: accounts of health and illness from East London*. London: Tavistock.

Daly, M., & Kelly, G. (2015). *Families and poverty: Everyday life on a low income*. Bristol: Policy Press.

Department for Communities and Local Government. (2011). *English indices of deprivation 2010*. London: DCLG.

Elliott, E., Harrop, E., Rothwell, H., Shepherd, M., & Williams, G. (2010). *The impact of economic downturn on health in Wales: A review and case study*. Cardiff School of Social Sciences Working Paper 134.

Geronimus, A. T. (2003). Damned if you do: Culture, identity, privilege, and teenage childbearing in the United States. *Social Science and Medicine, 57*, 881–893.

Goffman, I. (1963). *Stigma: Notes on the management of a spoiled identity*. New York: Simon and Schuster.

Graham, H., & McDermott, E. (2006). Qualitative research and the evidence base of policy: Insights from studies of teenage mothers in the UK. *Journal of Social Policy, 35*(1), 21–37.

Holland, J. (2009). Young people and social capital: Uses and abuses? *Young – Nordic Journal of Youth Research, 17*(4), 331–350.

Holstein, J., & Gubrium, J. (2008). *Handbook of constructionist research.* New York: Guilford.

Information Services Division. (2014). *Healthy life expectancy.* Scottish Public Health Observatory. Retrieved from http://www.scotpho.org.uk/population-dynamics/healthy-life-expectancy/key-points

Information Services Division. (2015). *Teenage pregnancy: Year of conception ending 31 December 2013.* NHS Scotland. Retrieved from http://www.isdscotland.org/Health-Topics/Maternity-and-Births/Teenage-Pregnancy/

Kingfisher, C. P. (1996). *Women in the American welfare trap.* Philadelphia, PA: University of Pennsylvania Press.

MacDonald, R., Shildrick, T., Webster, C., & Simpson, D. (2005). Growing up in poor neighbourhoods: The significance of class and place in the extended transitions of 'socially excluded' young adults. *Sociology, 39*(5), 873–891.

McNulty, A. (2010). Great expectations: Teenage pregnancy and intergenerational transmission. In S. Duncan, R. Edwards, & C. Alexander (Eds.), *Teenage parenthood: What's the problem?* London: Tuffnell Press.

Morgan, D. H. J. (1996). *Family connections: An introduction to family studies.* Cambridge: Polity.

Morgan, D. H. J. (2013). *Rethinking family practices.* Basingstoke: Palgrave Macmillan.

NOMIS. (2015). Official labour market statistics: Area profiles. Retrieved September 30, 2015, from https://www.nomisweb.co.uk/home/profiles.asp

Oakley, A. (1981). Interviewing women: A contradiction in terms. In H. Roberts (Ed.), *Doing feminist research.* London: Routledge and Kegan Paul.

Office for National Statistics. (2012). *Statistical bulletin: Conceptions in England and Wales 2010.* London: Stationery Office.

Office for National Statistics. (2013). *Regional labour market statistics, January 2013 release.* London: Stationery Office.

Office for National Statistics. (2014). *Life expectancy at birth and age 65 by local areas in England and Wales.* London: Stationery Office.

Office for National Statistics. (2014a). *Statistical bulletin: Births in England and Wales 2013.* London: Stationery Office.

Prior, S. (2011). Overcoming stigma: How young people position themselves as counselling service users. *Sociology of Health and Illness, 34*(5), 697–713.

Richards, H., & Emslie, C. (2000). The 'doctor' or the 'girl from the University'? Considering the influence of professional roles on qualitative interviewing. *Family Practice, 17*(1), 71–75.

Riessman, C. K. (1993). *Narrative analysis.* Newbury Park: Sage.

Riessman, C. K. (2008). *Narrative methods for the human sciences.* Thousand Oaks: Sage.

Riessman, C. K. (2011). What's different about narrative enquiry? Cases, categories, and contexts. In D. Silverman (Ed.), *Qualitative research*. London: Sage.

Scambler, G. (2004). Reframing stigma: Felt and enacted stigma and challenges to the sociology of chronic and disabling conditions. *Social Theory and Health, 2*, 29–46.

Scambler, G. (2009). Health-related stigma. *Sociology of Health and Illness, 31*, 441–455.

Scambler, S. (2012). Bourdieu and the impact of health and illness in the life-world. In G. Scambler (Ed.), *Contemporary theorists for medical sociology*. Abingdon: Routledge.

Scambler, G., & Hopkins, A. (1986). Being epileptic: Coming to terms with stigma. *Sociology of Health and Illness, 8*, 26–43.

Scambler, G., & Paoli, F. (2008). Health work, female sex workers and HIV/AIDS: Global and local dimensions of stigma and deviance as barriers to effective interventions. *Social Science and Medicine, 66*(8), 1848–1862.

Silverman, D. (2013). *Doing qualitative research*. London: Sage.

Stats Wales. (2013). Life expectancy by gender and year. Retrieved September 30, 2015, from https://statswales.wales.gov.uk/Catalogue/Health-and-Social-Care/Life-Expectancy

Strauss, A., & Corbin, J. (1990). *Basics of qualitative research: Grounded theory procedures and techniques*. Thousand Oaks, CA: Sage.

Taulbut, M., Walsh, D., Parcell, S., Hanlon, P., Hartmann, A., Poirier, G., et al. (2011). *Health and its determinants in Scotland and other parts of post-industrial Europe: The 'Aftershock of Deindustrialisation' study – phase 2*. Glasgow: Glasgow Centre for Population Health.

Thomson, R. (2009). Thinking intergenerationally about motherhood. *Studies in the Maternal, 1*(1), www.mamsie.bbk.ac.uk

Thomson, R., Bell, R., Holland, J., Henderson, S., McGrellis, S., & Sharpe, S. (2002). Critical moments: Choice, chance and opportunity in young people's narratives of transition. *Sociology, 36*(2), 335–354.

Tyler, I. (2013). *Revolting subjects: Social abjection and resistance in neoliberal Britain*. London: Zed Books.

Walsh, D., Bendel, N., Jones, R., & Hanlon, P. (2010). It's not 'just deprivation': Why do equally deprived UK cities experience different health outcomes? *Public Health, 124*(9), 487–495.

Wenham, A. (2015). 'I know I'm a good mum – No one can tell me different': Young mothers negotiating a stigmatised identity through time. *Families, Relationships and Societies*, doi:10.1332/204674315X14193466354732

Williams, F. (2004). *Rethinking families*. London: Calouste Gulbenkian Foundation.

4

'I was Scared but I was Happy': Getting Pregnant as a Teenager

In this chapter, we hear from the young people and their families for the first time as they begin to tell their stories. Taking a chronological approach to pregnancy and parenting, the chapter explores the experience of becoming pregnant, in particular the potentially challenging issue of telling other people, followed by the need to make decisions about the pregnancy.

Becoming pregnant can be welcome or unwelcome for anyone, teenager or older, depending partly on whether pregnancy was planned or unplanned. An unplanned or unintended pregnancy is not necessarily unwanted, and whilst the pregnancy itself may not be intended, a baby may be a welcome addition to the family. This chapter will discuss the complex feelings and decisions involved in the lead up to, and immediate consequences of, a teenager saying 'I'm pregnant'.

Some studies indicate that most teenage pregnancies are unplanned (for example, Anderson et al. 2007). However, our understanding of this is imprecise, not least because as Barrett and Wellings (2002) discuss, there is a great deal of ambivalence about the terms planned, unplanned, intended and unwanted. Teenagers may be particularly unlikely to use the terms planned and unplanned (Finlay 1996). Some evidence shows

© The Editor(s) (if applicable) and The Author(s) 2016
S. Brown, *Teenage Pregnancy, Parenting and Intergenerational Relations*,
DOI 10.1057/978-1-137-49539-6_4

that teenagers and women in lower-income groups are less likely to plan their pregnancies (Barrett and Wellings 2002; Family Planning Association 1999), and for teenagers this may be because of problems with contraception. These problems can stem from a number of, and indeed combination of, causes: a lack of knowledge about different methods and how to use them, a lack of knowledge about their own menstrual cycles (which are still developing and may not have settled into a regular rhythm), poor advice from medical professionals and contraceptive failure (see Pratt et al. 2014 for a useful systematic review of contraception and unintended pregnancy).

Barrett and Wellings discuss the idea of 'accidental' pregnancy, and Judith Green's work on the social construction of accidents (Green 1997) is illustrative here. The rational view of accidents is that they 'just happen' and therefore there is no blame attached; however, accidental pregnancy is regarded differently because an individual could, in theory, have chosen to act rationally (by obtaining and correctly using contraception) and therefore have avoided the accident (of conception). Green argues that in the modern world, it is often perceived that fate has no part to play, and that accidents have become predictable in terms of risk and chance, therefore becoming not a true accident, but a 'paradigmatic marker of a failure of risk management' (Green 1997, p. 141). In this context, given that most teenage pregnancies are unplanned, but contraception is free and widely available, teenage pregnancy becomes a clear and visible mark of failure. Dominant discourses of teenage pregnancy tend to focus on the unplanned nature of most teen pregnancies to the extent that they are often regarded as reckless and irresponsible. As Alldred says, 'Implicitly, and even explicitly in some hostile accounts, early motherhood is assumed to be the result of unsafe sex, in casual encounters, by young women who are not in an ongoing relationship and are precociously and promiscuously (hetero)sexual' (Alldred 2011, p. 141). However, given what we know about young people's difficulties with negotiating the use of contraception, and then using it successfully, taking this risk-based approach to understanding the situation is far from helpful. Several authors have argued that it is too simplistic an approach, ignoring the difficulties young women have in negotiating condom use (Hillier et al. 1998; Abel and Fitzgerald 2006) and the power imbalances in relationships which make it problematic for young women to be seen to be planning sex (Holland et al. 1990; Luker 1996). Public health discourses which emphasise the need for young women to develop self-esteem fail to acknowledge the dangers of assertiveness to an acceptable identity for young women (that is, in sexual terms, one who is passive, does not plan sex, and does not appear to desire sex) (Brown 2015), with the focus on self-esteem ignoring the social contexts of young people's relationships. Public health and health promotion messages often make unrealistic assumptions about 'the level of agency and control afforded to young people' (Shoveller and Johnson 2006, p. 48). Teenagers, therefore, are treading a very difficult path in negotiating relationships and their own reputations, knowing that any slip will not merely be seen as an accident, but a marker of their failure to behave rationally and manage their own risk. As we saw in Chapter 2, this risk-based thinking characterised the New Labour approach to the TPS, making assumptions that all teenage pregnancies were as a result of failure of one sort or another. Where evidence exists of teenage pregnancies being planned (Coleman and Cater 2006), there was condemnation of the research itself and insistence that pregnancy can never be a positive option for young people (BBC News Online 2006).

Geronimus (2003) has argued that in America, conventional wisdom is that early childbearing has disastrous consequences in terms of educational and occupational attainment, and in particular teenage parenting by African Americans violates a White American model of educational and occupational achievement. The implication, she argues, is that if only African Americans would adopt the nuclear family and delayed fertility norms of European Americans, this would result in social, economic and political equality. Similar arguments could be made in the UK in terms of class; the policy approach seems to be that if only teenage girls would be more middle class and less working class, social, educational and economic disparities would wither away. In addition to ignoring any structural disadvantages influencing people's lives, this model fails to acknowledge that in both the USA and the UK, women from working-class backgrounds or living in deprived neighbourhoods often do not see themselves as educational high achievers or as career women, motherhood and family being higher priorities for many than being a high earner. In addition, in many communities, being a high earner is unlikely to be an option for many young people. As one young (17-year-old) woman said, during the development work for an earlier study (Brown and Guthrie 2010):

> I didn't plan to have my babies just yet, but I find myself pregnant and it's either this or plucking chickens.

Therefore, where young women see their opportunities for meaningful and secure employment as being limited, motherhood becomes a good option.

The majority of research and policy documents about teenage pregnancy focus on young women, with young men either not featuring at all, or mentioned in passing. Where they do appear in the policy literature in particular, they are often portrayed in a negative light, with the focus being on the lack of support they provide to the mother, and their minimal involvement with their children (Ross et al. 2010). There is a growing body of research challenging these perceptions, in a similar manner to the growth of research that challenged commonly held assumptions about young women who become mothers (for example, Arai 2003, 2009; Duncan 2007; Duncan et al. 2010). This chapter begins to tell the stories of the young parents and parents-to-be, commencing with when they found out they were pregnant, and the impact this had. The appendix provides details about the individuals mentioned below; all names have been changed to maintain anonymity.

'I'm Pregnant'—Telling Parents

All the teenagers who took part in the interviews, and most of those who took part in the focus groups, had not planned to get pregnant. For some, the pregnancy resulted from contraceptive failure (for example, being unaware that sickness made the oral contraceptive pill less effective); a few described how they had been 'caught' while switching from one method to another, not realising that there might be a need for additional protection for a short time. Many young women struggle to find contraception that suits them (Jewell et al. 2000), and will switch from one method to another until they do. Those who had not been using contraception had either been 'caught in the moment' or had thought they could not get pregnant because previous unprotected sex had not resulted in a pregnancy, so they thought they were infertile. Hoggart and Phillips (2011) had similar responses in their study, while Coleman and Cater (2006) found that some young women who had not conceived after unprotected sex were afraid of finding that they were infertile. McDermott and Graham (2005) found that fear of telling parents about a pregnancy, and the parents' negative reaction, was common. In this study, because none of the interviewees had been trying to get pregnant, they were shocked and upset themselves, as well as being fearful of telling their parents:

> I cried and said my mum is going to kill me (laughs) and then I just didn't know what to do. (Zara)
>
> Scared, very scared. I don't know, it didn't seem real at the time, it seemed a bit—because I was shocked obviously. I was still only just kind of, just turned a teenager and was going out to party if you like, and then it was all over (laughs). (Naomi)

Several of the young women said that they were afraid of telling their parents, but also that they were worried about the reaction they would get from other people around them, beyond the family. Haley got pregnant when she was 16, and was 17 when her son was born:

Haley   It was the main fact that I was scared, scared about what people are thinking and everything.
SB   Were you worried about telling your mum and dad?
Haley   Yeah, so scared.
SB   Then how did they react?
Haley   My mam was well with it, but we'd just lost our nephew so my dad was really scared. He wasn't really happy with it.

Haley's older sister's four-month-old son had died shortly before Haley got pregnant, and two other nephews had died at a young age in the previous five years, so her father's reaction to her pregnancy was one of fear that having another grandchild would inevitably lead to another death. As a result, he had been withdrawn from Haley during her pregnancy, and as she said, 'I think I was about eight months when he started talking to me properly.' Later, Haley's mother Tina joined the interview, at a point at which Haley had said she knew that getting pregnant at 16 'wasn't the end of the world':

Tina   You were still scared to tell me though, weren't you?
Haley   Yeah, obviously.
Tina   Yeah, I don't know why, you were 16.
Haley   I know—but it's still awkward, isn't it?

Haley had not in fact told her parents directly. She told her sister, her sister told their mother Tina, and Tina told Kevin, their father. Early in the interview, Haley said that her mother 'was well with it' in her reaction to the pregnancy, and later on she said 'my mam loved it' that she was having a baby. However, a week previously when Tina had been interviewed alone, her reaction to my question about how she felt about Haley's pregnancy was quite different:

> Gutted, I was absolutely gutted.

She felt 'gutted' because Haley was the youngest of her three daughters and the third to become pregnant as a teenager, despite the efforts Tina had made to educate her about sex and contraception. Haley had been doing well at school, and Tina was like many of the parents in 'wanting better' for her daughter. However, following this initial reaction, she had then been very supportive, and again this captures the mixed feelings that although the pregnancy might be unplanned, a baby was not unwanted. As we shall see in Chapter 6, many of the grandparents and grandparents-to-be expressed joy at the arrival of new life and the next generation in the family; as Kirkman et al. (2001) found, parents who were unhappy about the pregnancy often became loving once their grandchild was born.

For some of the young women, someone else realised or suspected that they were pregnant before they did. Megan was 15 when her mother asked her if she was pregnant:

> My mother, she knew before I told her, because of my mood swings and the way I was crying a lot more and just not speaking to her like I would, trying to back off a bit. So she asked me, and I said no, and I burst out crying. And she said 'I've got a test here, I want you to go and take it.' ... I took it, I said

'mum I'm pregnant,' and I ran. I just ran and I didn't want to come back. And she just cried, she just cried and said 'Megan, I'm going to be here with you whatever you want to do', because obviously I was young, she said 'look, you can keep the baby, you don't have to keep the baby, just I'll be able to support you', and she did. And his family were the same, brilliant.

Megan had also been afraid of wider reactions, both those of her family and her boyfriend Owen's family, as well as people in the wider community. This was partly due to their very young ages. Megan was 15 when she got pregnant, 16 by the time her daughter Elen was born; Owen was 15, and one of Megan's concerns was that people would react badly because she was older than him:

> I was scared! Really scared! I felt as if the family wasn't going to take it the way which I was hoping them to, and I was thinking that my boyfriend's family, because my boyfriend was younger than me when I got pregnant with my daughter. And what people would think of me.

Deciding how to tell parents the news was a major challenge for the young women, particularly if they were worried about the reaction they would get. As we heard, Haley let her sister be the bearer of the news and, whereas Megan ran away after her announcement, Sarah avoided direct contact even in the way she told her mother Paula:

> I got a text telling me she was pregnant, not face to face. Then it took a while for Sarah to pick the phone up and then I just ranted, but I soon got over it. It was her age.

Having sent the message, Sarah then turned her phone off and stayed out of the house for the rest of the day, only turning her phone back on when she thought her mother might be calm. Paula, now 35, was 17 when Sarah's older brother was born. She described herself as 'shocked and upset' by Sarah's news, but her reaction was a combination of feelings not only about Sarah's age, but about her own experience and that of her son, who had become a father at 16:

> Obviously me being a young mum myself I know how difficult it is to cope financially, and obviously with her, well it is mainly her age and the finance

of it really, which is a concern, but I am over it now (laughs) … It's nice now I've got used to it, but it took me a while to get round to the idea because my son was 16 when his girlfriend first got pregnant. I was just as angry and upset with him as much as I was with Sarah, but his girlfriend's a bit older than him.

This combination of feelings, of anger, disappointment and being upset as an initial reaction, followed by acceptance, was common amongst the parents of the teenagers, as was a commitment to support the young person and the baby. Zara's mother Janet, who was 17 when Zara's oldest brother was born and 22 when Zara, her third child, was born, captures this mixture of feelings:

> I was disappointed and I let her know that I was disappointed, but at the same time I was always ready to support her and I don't think at any time, I didn't expect her to move out, you know, I think I would have been absolutely gutted if she had've done.

Not only did Janet not expect Zara to leave home, she said a number of times during both interviews that she did not want her to leave, and that she was glad to have her daughter and granddaughter living with her. The disappointment that Janet and other mothers expressed stemmed most often from parents wanting something better for their children; having had first-hand experience of the hardships of young parenthood themselves, they did not want their daughters to have the same experience. Some of the older generation of mothers had left home as a result of arguments with their fathers, in some cases being told to leave because they were pregnant, as in Paula's case. Paula's older sister had had a baby when she was 15, and had lived at home; when Paula got pregnant at 17, it was too much for her father:

> When I told my dad I was pregnant it was dad who said 'well you are moving out', but my mam wanted me to stay, but my dad after everything, going through everything with my sister and having a child and that, he wanted me, I'd have rather lived at home but he wanted—it was difficult but at the time my mum and dad weren't getting on that great anyway, they are divorced now, so I thought for the best just to, I don't know, to keep the peace between my mum and dad, so I did it.

Others, like Janet, had been living in hostels or staying with friends or relatives when pregnant or with a small baby. Although most of the older generations had not had such bad experiences, they still expressed similar concerns about the difficulties their daughters would face.

Debbie's mother Sheila, who was 15 when she had her first son, also captures one of the difficulties in negotiating the situation of having a pregnant teenager and having been in that same situation themselves:

> Well, there was nowt [nothing] I could really, I was a bit upset but I thought well, I can't really say nothing because I was underage when I had my first child, but I did want better for her but at the end of the day it's just summat you think well, you can't do nowt, can you?

This difficulty was also apparent in some of the paired interviews, Paula for example saying several times that she did not regret having her children, although she had wished for something different for herself as well as for them:

> You see, I don't want it to come across that I'm like saying to Sarah that I regret having her or her brothers or anything, I'm not saying that, because obviously there's only a year between Sarah and her older brother so I was still young when I had Sarah, but I don't, I don't regret ever having any of them, I just wish I'd have done things a bit different.

The delicacy of trying to say 'don't do as I did', without implying that having children young has been problematic, is highlighted in this exchange between Janet and Zara:

Janet   It took a while and a few bad decisions along the way [to get settled and in a nice house].
Zara   Thanks!
Janet   What?
Zara   Bad decisions along the way. I was a decision.
Janet   I didn't mean you! (laughs)

Although the tone was, on the surface, quite light-hearted, with both mother and daughter laughing, Zara appeared to feel hurt that she might be classed as a 'bad decision' by her mother, who went on to explain the difficult circumstances she had faced as a 17-year-old, being homeless and pregnant with Zara's oldest brother.

Where there were already problems in the relationship between the teenager and her parents, the announcement of a pregnancy unsurprisingly made those problems worse. Both Katy's parents (who had separated when Katy was young) disliked her boyfriend:

> I went to see her, I told her what had happened and yeah she, my mum wasn't happy. My dad, he wasn't happy, nobody really spoke to me. I was happy but I was also a bit down because I thought, in my head I thought I was losing my mum and my dad—because they hated my partner as well so—they really didn't like him, and I'd ran away to be with him when I found out I was pregnant.

Despite her fears about becoming estranged from her parents, she persisted in her relationship with her boyfriend, Pete, and resisted her mother's attempts to control her and break the relationship up:

> I ran away because when my mum found out she kind of, she was like 'you're never seeing Pete again' and all this ... she was trying to be really strict about him and put some ground rules down and I was like, 'mum I'm already pregnant so what, you know, what can happen?' and she was just like, 'well I don't want you to see him anymore' and I was like, 'well I will'.

While Katy's relationship with her parents deteriorated during her pregnancy, Sharon, who lived with her father, felt that pregnancy had brought them closer together:

> I think me being pregnant has helped me and my family get along, because I didn't really talk to my dad, he'd always be there if I needed anything or need to talk about anything, but I wouldn't, I'd go to my nan or my aunt. But now he's constantly checking I'm OK, and when he comes home from work or when I come home, he's asking 'you all right?' 'How you feeling, have you had something to eat?' 'Sit down, I'll make you a cup of tea.'

Sharon's older sister had also been a teenage mother, and their father had reacted to the news of that pregnancy in a way that had taken them all by surprise. Being a very protective father, according to Sharon, they had expected him to be furious, and 'chase [the boyfriend] down the road with his spade' when her sister went into the garden to tell him she was pregnant:

> They said they was having a baby and my dad went to bed, just stopped what he was doing and went to bed. … He didn't really say anything, he just went to bed. Then he just came down the next day and said 'right then, there's going to be a baby, better get you sorted somewhere to live' and that was it. And from that point he was a complete different person.

This practical approach was not uncommon, in that once a baby is on the way there is a sense that, as Sheila said above, there is 'nowt you can do' about the pregnancy, so the baby must be prepared for. This feeling that there is nothing that can be done also connects with decisions about whether to continue with the pregnancy, discussed further below.

Reactions Outside the Immediate Family

As we have heard, many of the young women were also worried about how people beyond their parents might react to the news of a pregnancy. Young mothers are aware of the stigma surrounding teenage pregnancy (Yardley 2008; Wenham 2015), and the negativity towards teenage pregnancy in the media is pervasive (Hadfield et al. 2007). Awareness of the dominant discourses around teenage pregnancy unsurprisingly gives rise to fears about the reactions young women may get from those around them.

Reactions to the young woman's pregnancy amongst wider family members were mixed. Paula's mother, who had been a teenage mother herself and had three daughters who had all been teenage parents (although also had two sons who had not), reacted calmly to news of her granddaughter Sarah's pregnancy:

> She took it better than me. My mam always says there's worse things than having babies, she took it better than me. (Paula)

In contrast, Katy's grandmother had not been pleased when she heard that Katy was pregnant, not least because she disapproved of Pete, as did

Katy's parents. However, having initially run away from home to be with Pete, Katy later moved in with her 'nana' during one of the break-ups with him:

> Oh, my nana was amazing, my nana, she didn't like it when I first got pregnant but from being pregnant she was brilliant, from accepting that I was pregnant and I was having this baby, she was brilliant.

Some of the young parents whose grandparents had reacted badly felt that this was due to different attitudes between the generations. Hannah, aged 17, and Jo, aged 16, had both been afraid of telling their parents about their pregnancies, but had found their parents more accepting than members of the older generations:

Hannah	My granddad weren't too happy about it at all, he was like 'oh she isn't going to keep it, is she?' and my mum's like 'well, actually she is.' But everybody else was fine, everyone was happy for me.
Jo	My gran was the same; she wouldn't even talk to me. Everyone else was fine about it, but my gran didn't even talk to me.
SB	Why do you think your gran and your granddad reacted that way?
Hannah	Because they're old and they don't get it.
Jo	Yeah, I don't think it was something that you did when they were young, yeah.
Hannah	It's just something that didn't really happen when they were our age.

Other grandparents had the same mixed reaction as parents had; Debbie's grandmother, Eileen, felt the same as Sheila, Debbie's mother:

> I was upset at first because I wanted a bit more for her but now we've got used to it.

This feeling of wanting more for their children than they had had themselves was common across the older generations, with Eileen saying the same in relation to her daughter Sheila, who had become a mother at the age of 15.

Some people experienced direct disapproval from friends, who made comments that are consistent with the discourse of pregnancy being a 'negative end point' (Hosie 2007, p. 334) for a teenager. For Patti, aged 16 when she became pregnant, it was because she was doing well at school until that point:

Patti   My friends were really disappointed in me when I found out I was pregnant.

SB   Why?

Patti   Because I was like, once again not trying to blow my own trumpet, I was a very high level student. I was predicted all As, and like four Bs, I was a very high level student.

Patti subsequently moved north to be with her boyfriend, and did not take her exams.

The negativity was not confined to young mothers. Dave and Jenny, a couple who were both aged 18 when they found that they were expecting a baby, had experienced comments from friends:

Dave   A lot of my friends said I wouldn't be able to do it, as soon as I told them—

Jenny   —They said your life's over and this stuff.

Dave   One of my friends said 'your life's over,' you know, saying all this stuff, and then since she's been born he's been like 'oh yeah, you've done real well.'

Hosie (2007) and Vincent and Thomson (2010) found that the response of young women's schools to pregnancy influenced whether or not a pregnant school-aged teenager was able to continue with her education. They focussed mainly on the reactions of the school staff, although the potential for bullying by other pupils was mentioned. Haley, aged 16, had tried to continue attending school, but a combination of bullying from peers and pressure from staff about her poor attendance due to illness meant she asked her mother to transfer her to the 'schoolgirl mums' unit:

> She went to school but then she started getting stress off people there because she was pregnant. (Tina, Haley's mother)

Having found out she was pregnant shortly after completing her GCSEs, Naomi returned to school in September to begin A levels, but left very quickly, as both she and her 14-year-old sister were bullied and called names. Both Skeggs (2004) and Tyler (2008) refer to the classed disgust of deviance in the way teenage mothers are regarded, but in these cases, it seems that the young women were targets of disgust from within their own social settings, particularly schools.

Breaking the News to the Father-to-be

As almost all the pregnancies were unexpected, the news came as a surprise to the young women's partners. How they reacted, after what was a shock for most of them, depended to some extent on the status of their relationship. The news also altered some of the relationships. For couples who were in an established relationship, the news could still be a shock; Naomi describes her partner Jamie's initial reaction:

> Well, his face went blank, and he went white, and I thought he was going to pass out (laughs).

Lewis and Suzi, both aged 19, have two children together, their first being born when they were 17; here, Lewis talks about feeling shocked at the news that Suzi was pregnant with their first child, but quite quickly after stating this, he asserts that he was happy about the news:

Lewis   Shocked, didn't know what I wanted to do about it. I felt like my life was going to be over (laughs).
SB   So you've got two now?
Lewis   Yeah, at the same time.
SB   So how old were you when your first one was born?
Lewis   I was 17.

SB   And how old were you?
Suzi   17.
SB   You were both 17, so feeling of shock, Lewis. Were you the same
       or did you—
Suzi   —Yeah.
Lewis Only for a little while and then I was happy about it.

In Debbie's case, her boyfriend Gavin had guessed that she might be pregnant before she had realised, and it was because he had said this that she bought a pregnancy test. Although as we saw above, her initial reaction had been to feel shocked and upset, Gavin reacted quite differently:

I did the test and told him and he was really happy.

For some young men, getting their partner pregnant can be proof of their masculinity, giving them the evidence they need to demonstrate that they are a successful heterosexual man (Kimmel 2008; Richardson 2010; Weber 2012). Steve was delighted to hear that his partner Ella was pregnant, as they had been trying for a baby:

Steve I was over the moon, I said I didn't fire blanks to everyone.
Ella   He did! He said to my mum 'oh it works, I'm a proper man.'

Weber (2012) discusses the challenges that young men have in negotiating masculine roles, whereby getting a girlfriend pregnant both signifies their manhood and labels them as sexually risky and feckless. Like the young men in her study, who position themselves in opposition to the stereotype by claiming that fatherhood makes them responsible and is based on love, Steve claims the pregnancy as proof of his masculinity, and later goes on to talk about the love he has for Ella and their son.

Some partners had mixed feelings about the news of the pregnancy. Sarah's boyfriend is five years older than her and already has a child with a previous partner:

I don't think he believed me, he was like real shocked, and then when I was talking to him face to face I don't think he wanted me to keep it in a way, but then he was happy, but he wasn't because of my age.

Nikki's partner also had mixed feelings, but as the relationship was unstable at the time of Nikki's pregnancy tests, this is unsurprising:

> I mean a week before I did the test, I actually did one and it said negative and he seemed a bit happy that it was negative, and then when I said it was positive again, he sort of gave me a reaction that I really didn't want. I got the feeling that he didn't want it but then once it had settled down and that, and a bit later on when I rang him again, he was fine. But he hasn't really seen her. Just before I found out I was pregnant, we split up and then we got back together again and then we split up again and that's it.

Whereas Nikki and a few other young women in the study had been experiencing cycles of splitting up and getting back together again prior to finding out about being pregnant, in some cases the news itself affected what had appeared to be a steady relationship, most often negatively. In Zara's case, which was at one extreme, she had been in a steady relationship when she got pregnant, but her boyfriend was opposed to her continuing the pregnancy:

> As soon as I told him [about the pregnancy] he wanted me to have an abortion and then from that there was just loads of trouble with him. We had to get the police involved.

She went on to describe how she had had to change her mobile telephone number and remove all her social media profiles due to his threatening behaviour. She had not seen him since the birth of her daughter and he had not expressed any wish to see the baby or be involved in any way.

In some cases, the father-to-be had accepted the pregnancy and expressed an intention to be involved but this had changed once the baby was born; Amy's relationship, which she had thought would continue, had ended when her son was born:

> He was alright with it, he was wanting to see him and stuff, but when he was born he didn't bother, so … (shrugs).

Conversely, Jo's boyfriend had disappeared at the point she told him she was pregnant, only to reappear several months later:

Jo   Mine just completely ignored me, he wasn't even, didn't even get in contact until she was about four, five months old, so he knew, he just didn't bother, didn't care.
SB   So, do you still have anything to do with him, does he see her?
Jo   Yeah, he does now yeah, he sees her like three times a week.

Although their relationship as a couple had ended, the continued involvement of Jo's ex-boyfriend in his daughter's life mean that they were managing a degree of co-parenting, which is not uncommon (Mollborn and Jacobs 2015). This type of relationship is discussed further in Chapter 5.

What Now?

Having discovered that they were pregnant, the teenagers had to decide what to do about it. Several studies in the UK (Jewell et al. 2000; Turner 2004; Coleman and Cater 2006) and the USA (Furstenberg 2007) have shown that the decision about whether to terminate or continue with the pregnancy is strongly related to social class and socio-economic position, with young women in areas of socio-economic deprivation much less likely to opt for termination than young women in more affluent areas. In addition, a teenager whose mother had been a teenage mother is more likely to continue with the pregnancy (Seamark and Pereira Gray 1997). A young woman who chooses to continue her pregnancy to term then has the options of keeping her baby or having her/him adopted. In the past, adoption was seen as a solution to the 'problem' of unmarried motherhood (Thane and Evans 2012), but trends in the numbers of babies adopted have been continuing steeply downwards for many years. This section of the chapter discusses how the young women reached their decision about continuing their pregnancy and keeping the baby.

Adoption

The possibility of having their baby adopted was only mentioned by two participants, although it was also discussed in one of the focus groups. Naomi explains how, having ruled out an abortion, she and her partner Jamie then considered adoption:

> I know I thought about [adoption] because obviously I don't agree with abortion for myself, it's fine for anyone else, that's fine, but then I thought I couldn't physically give birth and then not get to see or hold or keep this baby, but then watch someone else like drive away in effect with my baby. I couldn't do that.

This considering of options was carried out in the sense that they felt they needed to look at all possibilities and rule them out, rather than actively thinking that they would, in fact, give their baby up for adoption.

A lengthy discussion in the Seaborough focus group centred on a segment in a recently shown reality TV programme where two teenagers had given their baby up for adoption:

Jenny   They gave it to really good parents, and I think they're good parents because they did the most selfless thing that they could have, because they didn't want to, you could see it in their eyes, they were distraught about it but they lived in a caravan and they had no money and they had parents who were drug addicts and they wouldn't have been able to raise the baby. I mean they could have done a good job because they were good people but they wanted more for her … I think adoption is a selfless thing to do, to me, I couldn't do it, I don't know how you can give your child to somebody else but if you are doing it for the right reasons, I think it's amazing.

Helen   I think that's incredible. If I saw my child call someone else mum, that would break my heart, I wouldn't be able to do that, do you know what I mean, so if they were able to see that someone else would do a better job of raising their child than they could, I think they are really strong people to be able to do that.

Jenny draws attention to conflicting ideas about what it takes to be a good parent; on the one hand, she says that the young couple in the programme would not have been able to raise the baby because of their difficult situation: poor living conditions, no money, drug-addicted parents. But in contrast, they were 'good people' themselves, despite their own parents having problems, so would have been able to do a good job. The focus group participants expressed a great deal of admiration for the young couple who could put what they thought were the baby's best interests, to be raised by more suitable parents, ahead of their own, whilst all saying that it was not something they could do themselves.

Abortion

Although young women in areas where teenage motherhood is relatively common have been found to be anti-abortion (Tabberer et al. 2000; Arai 2003), the extent to which this is a firmly held pro-life stance in general, as opposed to something that was not for them personally, is unclear. Very few of the young people in this study were opposed to abortion in principle, only one saying, in one of the focus groups, that she was anti-abortion and then being supported by another participant:

Patti   One of my friends pulled me to the side and told me it would be OK if I had an abortion, it would be OK, and she'd go with me and everything. I told her I'm not doing it.

Mel   I just think that's wrong.

Patti   At the time I thought it was very wrong, I was very much anti-abortion … [but] there is a bigger picture. As much as having a child does not stop you living your life, it is extremely restricting, extremely restricting. It's the kind of restrictions that maybe some people can deal with; I'm not one of them.

Interestingly, Patti refers to herself as being opposed to abortion in the past tense, saying *at the time* she thought it was wrong, before going on to describe feeling very restricted by having a baby, and not being the sort of person who can cope with those restrictions.

Most young women were like Naomi, who would not want an abortion themselves but did not object to it in principle, and would not bar other people from having them:

He'd asked about an abortion but I explained to him that that wasn't right for me … he wasn't like saying to me 'go and get one, go and get one,' he suggested it like he suggested adoption and everything else. Then we discussed about it again, and when he saw the scan photo (laughs) he was over the moon as well, so everyone was all in one boat.

Although several couples, like Naomi and Jamie, had considered whether to have an abortion only to dismiss the idea, only Zara had come under pressure from her boyfriend to have an abortion. However, Katy had been pressurised by her mother to have an abortion, and had seriously considered it herself, attending the two appointments with the counsellor and the midwife before making her decision without her mother:

My mum wanted me to get rid of Josh, she didn't want me to have him, she came to the doctors with me and she set up a thing where I went to see a counsellor about having an abortion and I went to see my midwife so I had the two appointments, I just had to pick which one I was going to and which one I wasn't, in the end I went to them both and I made my decision from talking to the counsellor that I wasn't going to have an abortion … I did it on my own … it was something I thought I needed to do on my own, so my mum wasn't happy, and me and mum ended up getting into a big argument, like I got a smack across the face for being clever, and my nana said that she wanted to smack me across the face, but other than that it was all OK.

Some studies have found that deciding to continue with a pregnancy that has been unintentional is seen as the responsible thing to do; for example, Hoggart (2012) quotes a participant in her study saying essentially that if she was old enough to have sex then she was old enough to deal with the consequences. Carrying on with an unplanned pregnancy is seen as being responsible in terms of taking on new responsibilities as part of growing up (Thomson et al. 2003; Alldred and David 2010). In Zara's case that sense of taking on the responsibility for her actions is combined with a wider sense of family duty to have children; a close relative was unable to have a baby, and therefore Zara felt it would be wrong to have an abortion:

I wasn't 100 per cent sure was I, but then—because family members can't have children, I thought no, I've done this, it's now my responsibility to go through with this, plus I don't really believe in abortion anyway so (shrugs).

A sense of the wider family, and the young person's place in that family, also played a part in Haley's decision. Her older sister's son had died, aged four months, a few months prior to Haley's pregnancy, and her sister had been the first person Haley had talked to about being pregnant:

Tina   I think one of the decisions of you not getting an abortion was because of losing [baby]—

Haley   —yeah I told her that—

Tina   —just before that, and your sister was—

Haley   —can't get rid of a—

Tina   —when you did mention about having an abortion.

Haley   She said it was like a slap in the face to get rid of a healthy baby when she had just lost one.

Tina   It was. I don't agree with them.

Haley   Yes. That's why I never did. I don't agree with them. I think they're fine in certain stages, I can't say that I don't agree with them at all.

By 'certain stages', Haley meant that abortions were acceptable up to eight weeks, but she continued to express mixed feelings about abortion. She and her mother appeared to be in agreement when they were discussing the topic together. However, when talking without her mother present, Haley's ambivalence becomes more apparent:

> Yeah, I thought about an abortion, because I was at college. I was on the way to doing things and stuff, I didn't want anything to change. But then I thought about it properly and I knew I didn't want to, I think you know heart in heart if you want to or not.

She explained that she had been to the sexual health drop-in centre in the city centre and had been given an appointment for an abortion, but when she got home and told her sister, that was the point at which the comment about abortion being 'a slap in the face' had been made. Thinking about it 'properly' then appeared to involve being quite heavily influenced by her sister and having potential feelings of guilt about choosing to 'get rid' of a healthy baby when both her sisters had previously lost babies. Within the family there was a significant difference of opinion, though.

Tina asserted several times during both interviews that she was opposed to abortion in almost all circumstances. However, Haley's father Kevin had had a completely different reaction, based on his fears for Haley and their family experiences, having lost three boys very young:

Tina   Her Dad, straight away said get rid of it, because he had a nervous breakdown when the last baby died—
Haley   He couldn't go through it again.
Tina   —and he went 'I can't handle it, they only die anyway, get rid of it'. And, I dunno now, it was hard—but he couldn't get close to you during your pregnancy either, could he, not properly.
Haley   I think I was about eight months when he started talking to me properly.

The decision to continue with the pregnancy and keep the baby was, for some of the young women, a combination of opposition to abortion for themselves, and a sense that keeping the baby was the right thing to do. Zara saw it as the responsible way to deal with the consequences of her own actions, and for both Haley and Zara there was a sense in which they were making a decision that was broader than having a baby just for themselves; both saw themselves as taking a decision as part of the family, and keeping their baby was significant in making up for the loss of other babies, or the loss entailed by relatives being unable to conceive.

Some, like Katy, saw having a baby as an opportunity to turn their lives around. She had earlier described how she had two appointments, one to see a midwife and one to see a counsellor about having an abortion, and despite pressure from her mother to have an abortion, she had decided to keep her baby. Having not done well at school, dropped out of college and not having a clear idea of the direction her life was going in, having a baby became the 'something' she wanted to do with her life:

At the time I had quit college and all that, and I just thought what am I actually going to do with my life anyway? If I don't have him, what am I going to do? You know, and I didn't have nothing, there was nothing I wanted to do, I didn't know what I wanted in my life at all.

If, like Katy, Megan and a few others in the study, young women have not done well at school and are unsure of what to do with their lives, having a baby gives meaning and purpose. We will see in the next chapter how this can provide a turning point as they take on the responsibilities of becoming a mother.

Conclusions

All the interviewees were worried about telling parents that they were pregnant, and assumed that they would be upset or angry. They also feared reactions from others, whether known, such as at school, or unknown, by strangers in the street, and many young women reported overhearing critical comments or getting 'mucky looks'. Young women know from the moment that they decide to continue with a pregnancy that they are taking on a stigmatised identity, which incorporates stereotypes about life on benefits and being too young to cope. It also has a particular kind of public stigma (Scambler 2004, 2009) attached to it, which means strangers feel they are allowed to comment in public on the young women. This enactment of stigma will be discussed further in the next chapter in terms of judgemental attitudes towards young parents, but it begins with a visible pregnancy.

Thinking about the options, that is, whether to have an abortion, to adopt, or to keep the baby, had been a part of the decision-making process in choosing to become a parent, and partners and families had been influential. Adoption had not been seriously considered by any of the interviewees. They had all decided against abortion as being wrong for themselves, although acceptable for other people; the objection to abortion was that it was wrong for them, not wrong per se. Other studies (Tabberer et al. 2000; Arai 2003; Coleman and Cater 2006) have found that anti-abortion views are common in areas with high teenage pregnancies, but as a personal rather than political objection. The young women's parents, in all but one case, had supported their decision not to have an abortion.

For the most part, the parents of the teenagers had been disappointed at the news of their daughters' pregnancies, often because they had hoped that their daughters would not follow in their footsteps to become a teenage parent. They had themselves experienced the same reaction when they had become teenage parents, in that their parents had been disappointed. However, once they accepted the news, parents of teens were supportive (and as we shall see, those who remained unhappy during the pregnancy became accepting and supportive once the baby arrived), and this is one area where there is a difference between the generations. None of the youngest generation had been told to leave home as a result of their pregnancy, whereas two of the older generation had. Their experience of the hardships they had faced seems to have fed into them wanting better for their daughters; the older generations did not want their teenagers to become parents. In addition, some of the grandparents of the current teenagers had been unhappy about the news of the pregnancy, and the younger generation accounted for this in terms of differences in beliefs between older and younger generations.

All the young mothers interviewed for this study were the daughters of women who had themselves been teenage mothers, and in some cases their mother had also been a teenage mother. Some had siblings who had become parents as teenagers, so the context of the decision to become a parent as a teenager is one in which the young people already had examples around them of successful teenage parenting. However, the mothers of the teenagers had been very clear and insistent about the difficulties of young parenthood and the need to use contraception, hence their disappointment with the pregnancy, to some degree. The underclass thesis (Murray 1990) of a transmission of 'pathologised moral and cultural values' (Alexander et al. 2010, p. 136) transmitted between the generations does not explain the experience of the families in this study because the older generation wanted their children to avoid a pregnancy and 'do better' than they had. The teenagers themselves used evidence of successful teen parenting around them as proof that it was not 'the end of the world', and that finding themselves pregnant unintentionally was not a disaster, but something they could cope with. Being the child of a teenage mother did not encourage them to become pregnant, but seeing others manage as a young parent meant that they felt they could continue the pregnancy, keep the baby, and become a good parent themselves. The next chapter goes on to explore the next stage in the teenagers' lives: becoming a parent.

Appendix: Participants in Young Parent and Family Interviews and Focus Groups

Note: All names are pseudonyms
Interviewees

Name	Age	Baby	Baby's age	Location	Notes
Naomi	17	Jordan	4 months	Seaborough	Living together and
Jamie	18				planning to get married
Katy	18	Josh	18 months	Seaborough	Co-parenting with Pete but not in a relationship
Sarah	16	Pregnant		Seaborough	In a relationship with baby's father
Paula	35			Seaborough	Sarah's mum; first baby at 17
Zara	19	Ellie	4 months	Seaborough	Baby's father not involved
Janet	41			Seaborough	Zara's mum; first baby at 17
Amy	17		4 months	Seaborough	Mum had first baby at 15. Baby's father not involved
Haley	17	Riley	6 months	Seaborough	Baby's father not involved
Tina	37			Seaborough	Haley's mum. First baby at 14
Kevin	39			Seaborough	Haley's dad
Nikki	19	Louise	3	Seaborough	Mum had first baby at 19
Debbie	17	Pregnant		Seaborough	In a relationship with baby's father
Sheila	41			Seaborough	Debbie's mum. First baby at 15
Eileen	64			Seaborough	Sheila's mum
Mary	72			Seaborough	Eileen's sister. First baby at 17
Phil	43			Seaborough	Debbie's dad
Megan	20	Elen and Aled	2 and 4	Carville	First baby at 15, second at 17. Lives with partner Owen

Focus group participants

Name	Age	Baby	Baby's age	Location	Notes
Becky	18	Pregnant		Seaborough	Living together
Carl	18			Seaborough	
Jenny	19	Ava	8 weeks	Seaborough	Living together
Dave	20			Seaborough	
Sharon	17	Pregnant		Seaborough	Lives with dad and boyfriend
Zara	19	Ellie	4 months	Seaborough	
Faye	19		20 months	Seaborough	Co-parenting but not in a relationship
Helen	19		9 months	Seaborough	
Lisa	20		14 months	Seaborough	Lives with partner; expecting second child
Jade	18		2		
Steve	25	Scott	5 months	Milton	Living together
Ella	19			Milton	
Patti	18		18 months	Milton	Lives with partner
Mel	19		8 months	Milton	Baby's father not involved
Fiona	20		1	Norland	Living with mother; baby's father involved
Jackie	18		18 months	Norland	
Jane	20		5, 2 and 3 months	Norland	First baby at 16; married with 3 children
Vicky	18		1	Norland	Baby's father not involved
Steph	19		2 and 1	Norland	
Nicole	15		18 months	Norland	Living with Mark's
Mark	18			Norland	mum
Lloyd	19		2 and	Barton	Living together
Amy	19		6 months	Barton	
Tanya	18		3	Barton	Baby's father not involved
Jo	16		6 months	Barton	Baby's father sees her 3 times a week
Hannah	17		8 months	Barton	In a relationship with the baby's father

References

Abel, G., & Fitzgerald, L. (2006). 'When you come to it you feel like a dork asking a guy to put a condom on': Is sex education addressing young people's understandings of risk? *Sex Education, 6*(2), 105–119.

Alexander, C., Duncan, S., & Edwards, R. (2010). 'Just a mum or dad': Experiencing teenage parenting and work-life balance. In S. Duncan, R. Edwards, & C. Alexander (Eds.), *Teenage parenthood: What's the problem?* London: Tuffnell Press.

Alldred, P. (2011). 'How come I fell pregnant?' Young mothers' narratives of conception. *International Journal of Adolescence and Youth, 16*, 139–156.

Alldred, P., & David, M. (2010). 'What's important at the end of the day?' Young mothers' values and policy presumptions. In S. Duncan, R. Edwards, & C. Alexander (Eds.), *Teenage parenthood: What's the problem?* London: Tuffnell Press.

Anderson, S., Bradshaw, P., Cunningham-Burley, S., Hayes, F., Jamieson, L., MacGregor, A., et al. (2007). *Growing Up in Scotland: First research report on Sweep 1 findings of the Growing Up in Scotland study*. Edinburgh: Scottish Government.

Arai, L. (2003). Low expectations, sexual attitudes and knowledge: Explaining teenage pregnancy and fertility in English communities. Insights from qualitative research. *The Sociological Review, 51*(2), 199–217.

Arai, L. (2009). *Teenage pregnancy: The making and unmaking of a problem*. Bristol: Policy Press.

Barrett, G., & Wellings, K. (2002). What is a 'planned' pregnancy? Empirical data from a British study. *Social Science and Medicine, 55*, 545–557.

BBC News Online. (2006). Teenagers 'choosing motherhood'. Retrieved September 30, 2015, from http://news.bbc.co.uk/1/hi/health/5186614.stm

Brown, S. (2015). 'They think it's all up to the girls': Gender, risk and responsibility for contraception. *Culture, Health & Sexuality, 17*(3), 312–325.

Brown, S., & Guthrie, K. (2010). Why don't teenagers use contraception? A qualitative interview study. *European Journal of Contraception and Reproductive Health Care, 15*, 197–204.

Coleman, L., & Cater, S. (2006). 'Planned' teenage pregnancy: Perspectives of young women from disadvantaged backgrounds in England. *Journal of Youth Studies, 9*(5), 595–616.

Duncan, S. (2007). What's the problem with teenage parents? And what's the problem with policy? *Critical Social Policy, 27*(3), 307–334.

Duncan, S., Edwards, R., & Alexander, C. (Eds.). (2010). *Teenage parenthood: What's the problem?* London: Tuffnell Press.

Family Planning Association. (1999). *Misconceptions: Women's attitudes to planning and preventing pregnancy.* London: FPA.

Finlay, A. (1996). Teenage pregnancy, romantic love and social science: An uneasy relationship. In V. James & J. Gabe (Eds.), *Health and the sociology of emotion.* London: Blackwell.

Furstenberg, F. (2007). *Destinies of the disadvantaged. The politics of teenage childbearing.* New York: Russell Sage Foundation.

Geronimus, A. T. (2003). Damned if you do: Culture, identity, privilege, and teenage childbearing in the United States. *Social Science and Medicine, 57,* 881–893.

Green, J. (1997). *Risk and misfortune. The social construction of accidents.* London: UCL Press.

Hadfield, L. Rudoe, N. and Sanderson-mann, J. (2007). Motherhood, choice and the British media: Time to reflect. *Gender and Education, 19*(2), 255–263.

Hillier, L., Harrison, L., & Warr, D. (1998). 'When you carry condoms all the boys think you want it': Negotiating competing discourses about safe sex. *Journal of Adolescence, 21*(1), 15–29.

Hoggart, L. (2012). 'I'm pregnant … what am I going to do?' An examination of value judgements and moral frameworks in teenage pregnancy decision making. *Health, Risk and Society, 14*(6), 533–549.

Hoggart, L., & Phillips, J. (2011). Teenage pregnancies that end in abortion: What can they tell us about contraceptive risk-taking? *Journal of Family Planning and Reproductive Health Care, 2011*(37), 97–102.

Holland, J., Ramazanoglu, C., Scott, S., Sharpe, S., & Thomson, R. (1990). Sex, gender and power: Young women's sexuality in the shadow of AIDS. *Sociology of Health and Illness, 12*(3), 336–350.

Hosie, A. C. S. (2007). 'I hated everything about school': An examination of the relationship between dislike of school, teenage pregnancy and educational disengagement. *Social Policy and Society, 6*(3), 333–347.

Jewell, D., Tacchi, J., & Donovan, J. (2000). Teenage pregnancy: Whose problem is it? *Family Practice, 17*(6), 522–528.

Kimmel, M. (2008). *Guyland: The perilous world where boys become men.* Harper Collins: New York.

Kirkman, M., Harrison, M., Hillier, L., & Pyett, P. (2001). 'I know I'm doing a good job': Canonical and autobiographical narratives of teenage mothers. *Culture, Health and Sexuality, 3*(3), 279–294.

Luker, K. (1996). *Dubious conceptions: The politics of teenage pregnancy.* Cambridge: Harvard University Press.

McDermott, E., & Graham, H. (2005). Resilient young mothering: Social inequalities, late modernity and the 'problem' of 'teenage' motherhood. *Journal of Youth Studies, 8*(1), 59–79.

Mollborn, S., & Jacobs, J. (2015). 'I'll be there for you': Teen parents' co-parenting relationships. *Journal of Marriage and Family, 77*(2), 373–387.

Murray, C. (1990). *The emerging British underclass*. London: IEA.

Pratt, R., Stephenson, J., & Mann, S. (2014). What influences contraceptive behaviour in women who experience unintended pregnancy? A systematic review of qualitative research. *Journal of Obstetrics and Gynaecology, 34*, 693–699.

Richardson, D. (2010). Youth masculinities: Compelling male heterosexuality. *British Journal of Sociology, 61*(4), 737–756.

Ross, N. J., Church, S., Hill, M., Seaman, P., & Roberts, T. (2010). *The fathers of children born to teenage mothers: A study of processes within changing family formation practices*. Glasgow: Children First.

Scambler, G. (2004). Reframing stigma: Felt and enacted stigma and challenges to the sociology of chronic and disabling conditions. *Social Theory and Health, 2*, 29–46.

Scambler, G. (2009). Health-related stigma. *Sociology of Health and Illness, 31*, 441–455.

Seamark, C., & Pereira, G. D. (1997). Like mother, like daughter: A general practice study of maternal influences on teenage pregnancy. *British Journal of General Practice, 47*(416), 175–176.

Shoveller, J., & Johnson, J. L. (2006). Risky groups, risky behaviour, and risky persons: Dominating discourses on youth sexual health. *Critical Public Health, 16*(1), 47–60.

Skeggs, B. (2004). *Class, self, culture*. London: Routledge.

Tabberer, S., Hall, C., Prendergast, S., & Webster, A. (2000). *Teenage pregnancy and choice. Abortion or motherhood: Influences on the decision*. York, UK: Joseph Rowntree Foundation.

Thane, P., & Evans, T. (2012). *Sinners? Scroungers? Saints? Unmarried motherhood in twentieth century England*. Oxford: Oxford University Press.

Thomson, R., Henderson, S., & Holland, J. (2003). Making the most of what you've got? Resources, values and inequalities in young people's transitions to adulthood. *Educational Review, 55*(1), 33–46.

Turner, K. M. (2004). Young women's views on teenage motherhood: A possible explanation for the relationship between socio-economic background and teenage pregnancy outcome? *Journal of Youth Studies, 7*(2), 221–238.

Tyler, I. (2008). Chav mum, chav scum: Class disgust in contemporary Britain. *Feminist Media Studies, 8*(1), 17–34.

Vincent, K., & Thomson, P. (2010). 'Slappers like you don't belong in this school': The educational inclusion/exclusion of pregnant schoolgirls. *International Journal of Inclusive Education, 14*(4), 371–385.

Weber, J. B. (2012). Becoming teen fathers: Stories of teen pregnancy, responsibility, and masculinity. *Gender and Society, 26*(6), 900–921.

Wenham, A. (2015). 'I know I'm a good mum – No one can tell me different': Young mothers negotiating a stigmatised identity through time. *Families, Relationships and Societies*, doi:10.1332/204674315X14193466354732

Yardley, E. (2008). Teenage mothers' experiences of stigma. *Journal of Youth Studies, 11*(6), 671–684.

5

'I wouldn't Swap It for the World': Being a Young Parent

Becoming a parent is both joyful and stressful for many people, of whatever age. The delight of a new baby combines with the tiredness of caring for them, the changes to relationships, and for women who were working before a baby was born, a change in role and perhaps in perceived status. These pressures and challenges are often assumed to be harder for young mothers to deal with due to their age, leading to fears about whether they will be able to cope. However, as Graham and McDermott (2006) point out, there is a contrast between quantitative and qualitative research findings on teenage pregnancy and parenting. Whereas quantitative research, which is predominant in policy formation, presents teenage pregnancy and parenting as almost unremittingly negative, qualitative research presents a more positive, as well as a more nuanced, picture. Indeed, whereas quantitative research points to teen parenting as a route to social exclusion, qualitative research shows how it can be a route to social inclusion.

Despite some positive images of teenage parents, for example, an exhibition of photographs at the Houses of Parliament in January 2015 which was accompanied by an article in The Guardian newspaper (Moorhead 2015), they are outweighed by negative portrayals in the media and in

© The Editor(s) (if applicable) and The Author(s) 2016
S. Brown, *Teenage Pregnancy, Parenting and Intergenerational Relations*,
DOI 10.1057/978-1-137-49539-6_5

policy. Studies in the UK, Australia and Canada have shown that young mothers are aware of the overwhelming cultural narratives about them (Leese 2014), but reject the negative stereotypes (Clarke 2013) and construct positive identities that outweigh them (Kirkman et al. 2001; Rolfe 2008). Many young mothers have been criticised in public, either directly or by overhearing remarks about them (Yardley 2008). Their response to the stigmatising negative images is to distance themselves from the stereotype by working hard to create and present an identity as a 'good mother' (Romagnoli and Wall 2012; Wenham 2015). Presentation of an identity is important particularly where the audience is a professional one (Leese 2014), not least because of the construction of young mothers as being at risk and therefore in need of surveillance (Romagnoli and Wall 2012; Breheny and Stephens 2007).

This chapter explores what it means for young people to become a parent and how they adapt to their new role. It considers how they feel about themselves as parents in the context of the negative discourses that surround them, their responses to the stereotypes, and their construction of their new lives and selves.

Becoming a Young Parent

As has been noted, much of the literature on teenage parenthood pays much more attention to young mothers than young fathers, not least because of the way young fathers and mothers are problematised in different ways. In this study, more young women than men took part, due mainly to the way they were engaged with the study, so that young men tended only to take part in the study if they were still in a relationship with the mother of their baby, and she had decided to take part and to ask them to join in. Hence in this chapter, the voices of young women outnumber those of young men, but this is partly a reflection of the balance between those who had remained a couple, and young women who found themselves parenting single-handedly. Nevertheless, young men's views have been included as much as possible, as well as the views of young women about the young fathers, in an attempt to include a broad perspective on being a young parent.

For some of the young women, deciding to become a parent was a choice they made because they felt unsure of what else to do in life, and that having a baby was a good option in the circumstances. Although all but one of the young women interviewed had not chosen to get pregnant, as discussed in the previous chapter, they had made conscious decisions about keeping the baby and becoming a mother. In other words, although they might not have chosen to get pregnant, they had chosen to become a mother. Katy had earlier described how she had two appointments, one to see a midwife and one to see a counsellor about having an abortion, and despite pressure from her mother to have an abortion, she had decided to keep her baby. As we heard in Chapter 4, she felt that having not done well at school, dropped out of college and not having a clear idea of the direction her life was going in, having a baby became the 'something' she wanted to do. Similarly, Megan was unsure about her future, and having changed schools then felt she had chosen the wrong subjects:

I've never known what I wanted to do when I was older, never known, I never had nothing set, and when I was in my GCSE year, I was in Carville High School and I took the wrong subjects and I wasn't happy with the subjects I took, it wasn't me.

For those young women who did not know what they wanted to do, becoming a mother could not only be fulfilling in itself, but also help them to develop confidence in themselves. Megan had discussed being treated for depression, but felt that having her children as an incentive to go out and to meet new people had helped her:

Since I've had the kids, I've been more, I'll go out, I'll meet new people, they've all got young kids so you'll go together for walks along the park, like into the park. I'm more doing stuff, to help me and the kids, because I get very depressed if I'm stuck in the house a lot, so I like to be out. So I find that the advantages are that it's helped me to be more confident in myself and with my kids.

For most of the young fathers to be, as their partners' pregnancies had been unintended, they had not made a deliberate choice to become a father; however they had, according to their partners, been pleased at the prospect. For Steve, meeting his partner Ella had brought about a change in the way he wanted to live his life:

> It weren't Scott that made the difference; it was meeting Ella that made the difference, it made me feel like—I'm actually wanting to settle down with her and stuff, so. Started just spending a lot of time with Ella instead of my mates I used to hang around with, and we got him so … (shrugs and smiles).

Although Steve says the birth of his son had not by itself prompted his desire to change, he had wanted to settle down with Ella and she got pregnant soon after they got together. Having a new family and a woman he loved had given him the incentive to avoid his previous associates, with whom he had got into trouble; Steve had been in prison, but said now that he had Ella and Scott, he had no intention of being in that situation again. In this sense, he is using a 'redemption script' (Maruna 2001). They planned to move away to make a new start, and were due to get the keys to their new house the week after the focus group.

One young father, Pete, (who was not interviewed) was described as actively wanting to become a father, to the extent that he had persuaded his then girlfriend, Katy, to have a baby. Although earlier she had described how becoming pregnant had enabled her to re-evaluate her life, and that having her son had meant that she felt she had turned her life around, her feelings at the beginning were ambivalent at best:

> When I got pregnant I didn't want Josh, not that I didn't want Josh, I didn't want to have a baby, but I kept him and obviously I wouldn't change it for the world now, but Pete was always the one that wanted me to get pregnant and wanted that life and wanted that family.

Katy and Pete had had a tempestuous relationship, and had split up and got back together several times including during the pregnancy:.

> I don't think we've been in a relationship for a maximum of a month since Josh has been around, since he was born. We got back together after he was born and then we broke up again, then we tried again like last year, it lasted

like five days and we've both said from there it's just never going to work between me and him, there's too much history with us and there's too much to try and forgive. Me and Pete have always been better as friends than what we ever have been in a relationship … he's a brilliant dad, worst boyfriend in the world but he's a brilliant dad.

Despite their unsettled relationship, Pete continued to be very involved in his son's life, caring for him several times a week. As Mollborn and Jacobs (2015) found in their study of teenage parents in Colorado, USA, co-parenting arrangements can continue after the end of a romantic relationship between the young couple, with many fathers wishing to remain involved with their child. Like the parents in Edin and Kefalas' study, 'being there' for the child was seen as important by both mothers and fathers. However, Pete was somewhat unusual in the context of this study. For most of the young women who were raising their children as single mothers, their former boyfriends had more sporadic contact with their children than Pete has with Josh.

The social context for many of the young people in this study is one where having a family by one's early twenties is both normal and desirable, and welcomed by the wider family. As Kirkman et al. (2001) found, families often welcome a baby even though they might not have welcomed the pregnancy. In Leese's (2014) study, the young mother who best managed the transition to motherhood had experience of caring for younger children in her wider family, and had a reference group (Shibutani 1955) of other people in her family who had become parents under the age of 16. Similarly, Debbie had helped her cousin and other relatives care for their young children, and had several other relatives including her mother, Sheila, and her great-aunt, Mary, who had become pregnant as teenagers. The Jones family, talking about their reactions to Debbie's unexpected pregnancy, also mentioned other family members; Mary, Debbie's great-aunt, talked about her happiness at hearing that her granddaughter was pregnant:

My granddaughter, she's having one, there's only eight weeks between her and Debbie. She's 20 and when she rang me I said 'Oooh!' (laughing) I said, 'I'm over the moon!'

The young women in this study had a reference point, in that their own mother had had her first child as a teenager, and many had a larger reference group within their family; Haley, who got pregnant when she was 16, had two older sisters, both of whom had had babies whilst teenagers, and Haley's mother Tina had had the first of her children when she was 14. Similarly Sarah, who was pregnant at 15, has an older brother who had had his children, twins, when he was 16, Sarah's mother Paula had had him when she was 17, both Paula's sisters had been teenage mothers, and each sister had a daughter who had been a teenage mother. Paula's mother had the oldest of Paula's sisters when she was 18, but unlike Paula and Sarah, was married. Some commentators may see this as evidence that there is an underclass somehow transmitting teenage pregnancy through the generations, as if it was a contagion passed from mother to daughter. However, although there is undoubtedly a connection between the generations in terms of becoming parents at a young age, the connection is less likely to be causal than cultural, in the sense of family, community and class cultures. The teenage mothers in Kirkman et al.'s (2001) Australian study did not interpret their family history of teenage pregnancy as a determinant of their pregnancy, but having a family story of success provided an alternative to the 'doom' narrative. Both Tina and Paula had raised their children with an awareness of the hardships of being a teenage parent, and told them about sex and contraception:

> I've always talked to them and told them how hard it was, and that—I don't regret any of my children but I wish I'd waited, do you know, like, lived life a little bit. (Paula)
>
> I told them everything, they knew everything about sex, condoms, you name it, and we were really open with them. But it happened, and she knew all about condoms, you name it. (Tina)

The fact that the young women had all been afraid to tell their parents about their pregnancy, and worried about the reaction they would get, suggests that they did not feel it was an acceptable course of action, still less encouraged. That the parents expressed disappointment, and said that they wanted something better for their daughters, suggests the same.

In the past, transitions to adulthood in many working-class communities followed a path of leaving school at 16 or 18, getting an apprenticeship or a job, and settling down, with early marriage and childbirth the norm. University attendance was and still is rare in the places where this study was conducted, although almost all the young people in the study were at college doing vocational courses, or intended going back to an interrupted college course. So, for many, becoming a parent at 17 or 18 is only a few years earlier than they would have planned to do it anyway. As Phoenix argued, delaying motherhood may make little sense to young working-class women with limited opportunities (Phoenix 1991), and as SmithBattle suggests, 'when few options exist, mothering is not viewed as a precocious event but as a pathway to adulthood that provides meaning and purpose' (2007a, p. 410).

Some of the young women expressed a wish that they had waited, but even those who said that would not have waited long. Asked if she would change anything about being a mother, Naomi, aged 17, replied:

> If I could do it a year or two ahead, but that's it, as long as I've got him exactly the same, exactly the same house.

Paula, aged 35, and mother of three children, had said that she wished she had waited, but then described the compensations of having had her children young, including having the energy to care full-time for a baby that she did not feel she had now, although she did care for her grandchildren, her son's two-year-old twins:

> Looking back at I said I wish I'd had waited, and I wish I'd done things differently, but seeing that now I've become a nana to twins, and I look after them on a weekend to give them a break and I do a lot for them, I'm glad I had mine young in a way, because I don't think I'd have [youngest son, 13], he's tiring and I don't think I could have him at my age now, I think I had more patience and more energy … I think in a way that's a good side of it. I think you are closer when you have your children young.

The right age to have a baby was most commonly said to be when one was in one's early twenties:

Twenty-three or 24. I think it's just early, but not too early, it's not old. (Haley)
   I think around about the age of 20-odd, it's more natural to have kids at that age. (Megan)

It was also felt that it was possible to be too young, in which case Paula suggests that the baby should be brought up by the grandmother:

I think 18's acceptable, 16 I think is young obviously, but I think you've got your own mind to know what you want, and anything below that I don't, I think maybe the mother should take over, I know that it's not their choice to have children but that is definitely a child bringing up a child isn't it?

Naomi cites a case of someone she knows doing just that:

We know a girl who was 14 when she had hers, and that was my little sister's age and I thought Jesus, my little sister would have no chance, she can't even look after a fish! But she lives with her mum, and she's still at school … but her mum has always got the baby.

Part of the concern about being the right age to become a parent was connected to ability to parent; as both Paula and Naomi indicate, there is a point at which a young woman could be considered too young and in many cases her mother, that is, the baby's grandmother, may well take over the role of raising the child. If the grandmother had been a young mother, she may be becoming a grandmother at a point when she has small children and may still be having children herself. As we heard in Chapter 3, inspiration for this study came from Lydia, one of the participants in a previous study (Brown and Guthrie 2010) who described how she had had her baby when she was 15, at which point her mother was 34, having had her first child, Lydia's older brother, when she was 15. Now in a new relationship, she had had a baby eight months before her grandchild was born. For Lydia, this had worked out well, as her mother looked after both young children which enabled her to return to college and complete her education.
   Paula captures the possible differences in attitudes to the right age to have a baby, based on educational aspirations and attainment:

I wonder, if you know people who've had babies young, you look at them and think, 'well, they did it so I can'. And I think the other thing is there is quite a big, or there seems to me to be a big split these days, in that girls who go off to university and have careers and all that, there was a thing in the paper only the other day, they are waiting until they are in their thirties and even their forties to have babies.

This is closely tied to class, as Jewell et al. (2000) found in their study, where the group they described as 'disadvantaged' thought that the best age to start a family was between 17 and 25, whereas the 'advantaged' group put a greater emphasis on university and career and thought a good age would be late twenties or early thirties. Working-class girls are also more likely to have experienced other family members having children young, as well as other young women in their school and community. In contrast, middle-class girls are more likely to have been encouraged by the parents to go to university, and to have less experience of close family with young children. As Paula suggests, there is a growing class-related age differential in age of mother at the first birth of her baby; education is linked with later and less childbearing, with 'increasing divergence in family and working lives between women who have post-compulsory education and those who do not' (Smith and Ratcliffe 2009, p. 41). In addition, in many industrialised countries including the UK, there is a trend for delayed motherhood as more women are employed (Hansen et al. 2009), which will contribute to a widening gap between typical age at first birth for working class women compared to middle-class women.

Although several participants had views about a good age to have a baby, Steve sums up the views of many about there not being a right age to have one, referencing the media prevalence of negative stories about young parents:

> Papers saying young parents can't cope and stuff, you should wait until you're in your thirties to have kids and stuff. I think it's all irrelevant; you should have a kid when you feel like you're ready to have a kid.

One of the key differences between the generations in terms of parenting relates to marriage. As stated earlier, in the past the problem of young motherhood related more to the marital status of the mother than to her age, and in many cases this 'problem' was solved by marriage. Mary had her first baby in 1958, when she was 17, and although he was conceived before she was married, by the time he was born she had married his father, her first and only boyfriend:

> Oh, I was married when he was born, because them days, it was a privilege of a man to marry you, well morally, but my husband was in the forces when I had my eldest but I lived with his mam, so she helped me to bring him up.

Despite Mary getting married, her brother had expressed his disapproval of her situation:

> My husband was my first boyfriend I met, to say we got married like, and my brother said 'I think it's disgusting', and my mam just said to him, 'well it's one of those things'. Like I said to Debbie, 'you're not the first and you won't be the last', but you know, he was alright after that.

Mary's mother's acceptance of the pregnancy outside marriage being 'just one of those things', and her mother-in-law's help and support with raising her new baby while her husband was away in the army, meant that Mary did not feel stigmatised by being a young mother, not least because she had done the right thing by getting married. From her knowledgeable and experienced position, she was able to offer Debbie, her great-niece, the same support and acceptance that she had experienced.

Mary and her sister Eileen went on to talk about having to get married, and it not being allowed for unmarried couples to sleep together, despite us having just discussed Mary and her husband conceiving a baby before they were married:

Eileen   Like you had to, you didn't have to get married but it was a thing where you knew you had to, you couldn't have a baby out of wedlock, put it that way.

Mary   And they didn't believe in living together like they do in today's world.

Eileen   You daren't sleep together, that wasn't allowed, but it has changed completely.

Certainly in the 1950s and into the 1960s there was a very strong pressure for young couples to be married by the time a child was born, if that child had been conceived out of wedlock (the couple having a so-called 'shotgun marriage'). In that sense, a dramatic shift has taken place in attitudes, in that people no longer feel the need to be married, and social pressure to get married seems to have lessened. However, for several of the young couples, marriage was something they wanted and were planning to do:Naomi: We want to get married as well because—it's going to be really sloppy this, on your recording! (laughs) But I couldn't feel for anyone else and I don't think he could—or he better not!

Jamie	Like as well, if you say 'me and my girlfriend have got a baby', it sounds more childish whereas if I say 'me and my fiancée' or 'my partner', you sound more mature and steady and I think it shows that we are serious about it, that we are stable.
Naomi	But then it's not just for everyone else's benefit so anyone else thinks that we're stable, it's for ourselves.

Jamie and Naomi were both very conscious of the impressions that other people had both of themselves and young parents in general, and talked about appearing smartly dressed, with a well-dressed and well-cared-for baby in order to counter potential accusations about being a bad parent. It is interesting to note, therefore, that Jamie wants to be married partly as a public demonstration of how stable he and Naomi are.

Becky	I want to get married. We want to get married, don't we? It's just expensive.
Carl	It costs a bomb.
Becky	It's something for the future, isn't it? I'm writing a list of things, because I think it's important to be married. I think that moral has gone out the window but I like the old-fashioned way. I like the dating and the courting and getting to know each other.

Becky's motivation for getting married came from a strong moral sense of what was right in terms of relationships and stability. Having experienced a great deal of instability in her life, including trying to look after her four younger siblings to keep them out of care, and having a mother who was a drug addict, much of what she expressed during the focus group discussion related to her desire to be settled and stable, with her own house that she could decorate as she chose.

However, instability in childhood did not necessarily lead to a desire to get married to find stability themselves; whereas Becky had experienced a disrupted childhood, both Jamie and Naomi had very stable family backgrounds. Not all young couples expressed a desire to get married, although those who were in stable relationships either already lived together (Jenny and Dave, Megan and Owen, for example) or planned to get a house together (Debbie and Gavin, Sarah and Darren).

The teenage parents had grown up with a range of experiences of their parents' marital and relationship histories. Sarah's mother Paula had been in a relationship with her partner since she was 16 and he was 18, and they had three children together, but had not married. Debbie's mother Sheila also had three children with her partner, and they got married between the births of their first and second children, Debbie's older brothers. Tina had had her first child when she was 14, and no longer had any involvement with the father. She had married Haley's father before the birth of their first child together, Haley's older sister, and they had three children together. In these families, whether or not marriage had taken place, there is a great deal of stability in terms of the children's upbringing, and this, as discussed later, has contributed to the belief expressed by several of the teenagers that having children young is not the end of the world.

Other young parents had less stable backgrounds. Zara's mother Janet had experienced domestic violence and homelessness after leaving her father's home to live with her boyfriend at the age of 16, when she was pregnant, and then leaving the father of her two sons when she was pregnant with the second due to his violence. She married Zara's father before Zara was born, but he was also violent, towards Janet and Zara, and that relationship ended in divorce.

Katy described her mother as 'putting men first' and described a series of relationships following the separation of her mother and father which had resulted in several house moves and changes of school for Katy:

> She follows her heart a lot, and she did move us [ten miles away], and that kind of messed up my schooling and stuff because they were on a higher level there, and then we came home. And then we did move to Scotland because my mum fell in love again, then we came home again.

In contrast, after the end of his relationship with Katy's mother, her father had met and married a woman who Katy referred to as her step-mother. Katy's history led her to declare that she did not want to be like her mother, and did not want her son to think about her the way she thought about her mother. In particular, she planned to stay single and not introduce 'a series of boyfriends' to her son, in case he became fond of them and they then left.

There is no clear pattern, therefore, in the way the teenagers' experiences of their parents' relationships have influenced their views of marriage and relationships, although the common thread they all share is a wish for stability. For some, like the couples wishing to get married, stability comes in the form of marriage; for others, like Katy, stability is achieved by staying single and not allowing relationships with men to disturb the upbringing of her son.

Being a Mother

Although few of the young women had intended to become mothers, at least not for a few years, they were all determined to be a good mother, and despite acknowledging the hardships and challenges, Naomi's feelings are typical:

> I just love it all, I wouldn't swap it for the world! (laughs)

Similarly, Katy talked at length in both her interviews about the difficulties she and the father of their young son had experienced, not the least of which was that Pete (her former partner) had gone on to have a son with another partner, but said she would be selective about what she would change, if she could:

> I wouldn't change it now for the world. I'd maybe change the stuff that me and Pete have gone through but I wouldn't change Josh for the world.

Asked about what were the best things about being a mum, Katy replied, 'I don't really know.' She went on to say:

> I get really, really lonely … so I don't know, there isn't really a best bit, it's just kind of constant, you know, there is hard times when, like, you know, like obviously when I've got no money or anything … No, I wouldn't say there is a best bit.

But having said that there 'isn't a best bit', and that sometimes her life is hard, she went on to be quite positive:

> I'd say this is all quite good that, you know, obviously being in the paper and having a job now is all brilliant but, you know, in the end it is kind of just about me and Josh.

Nikki had a great deal of pride in her daughter, which meant she could say that for her, motherhood was 'brilliant':

> It's just brilliant, all them bits like coming up saying 'mummy I love you', I can have a really hard day and she's like 'mummy I love you', it makes me cry. Seeing how good she's getting on, like in nursery they keep moving her up rooms early because she's so clever. But yeah, just like all the moments where she comes up, 'I love you', and the way she is getting on and thing like that, the way I can see her blossoming into a really intelligent child, they're the best bits.

Some of the young parents had moved out of their parental homes; Naomi and Jamie, and Megan and Owen, now had their own homes and for both Naomi and Megan, their role as parents also meant they were now managing their own households. Having said that 'it's nice knowing that at my age I can do all', Naomi went on to detail what she felt were her responsibilities for the household and family as a whole:

> The hardest bit is just making sure everything is right, every one's happy, and obviously because I'm the mother I get put in charge if you like, because we all know that women, not to be sexist but women take care of the kids, don't you? But the hardest bit, like I say, is keeping the house all intact, keeping him [the baby] intact (laughs), and keeping his dad happy. Everyone has got to be happy, I've got to be happy myself as well, so, but that's the hardest bit (pause). And I mean that's not that hard, but that's the hardest bit, so everything else has got to be swimming and good.

Having put her son and her partner first, Naomi acknowledges that she needs to be happy too, but clearly shoulders the burden of responsibility for her family in terms of caring. What is striking is how Naomi acknowledges the gendered nature of her role ('not to be sexist but …') but accepts it anyway, seemingly without question: as the mother, she is in charge of the home and the well-being of the whole family. Most of the young people talked about roles within the family in this traditional gendered way, women as home-makers, men as providers and breadwinners; even where they were not necessarily fulfilling this role themselves, they presented it as the desirable norm.

Megan had decided to move into her own house because she felt she needed independence, as a parent, from her own parents:

> It was a big step, it was, like though I'd rather, because I was, I'm the type of person I'd rather have my own space. And it was easier for me to do stuff as myself as a young mother, to help Elen, than having my parents trying to tell me what to do and, you know. But yeah, I found it all right.

She was aware that people within her community were talking about her:

> People were like when I had Elen, 'I wonder if she's going to cope', and 'how is she going to do it like with the money, she hasn't got a job or nothing?' But I found it all right, you know, I found it all right. I did get the odd day when I was like, 'God, I haven't got money to go to town or nothing', but as long as Elen had nappies, as long as I had gas and electric in the house.

It was often not enough for the young parents to feel they were managing well; they also felt under pressure to prove themselves to be good parents to outsiders.

Negotiating a Stigmatised Identity

Several studies have found that teenage mothers are aware of their position as a member of a stigmatised group (Rolfe 2008; Yardley 2008), and the young parents in the study were all aware of social perceptions that their age meant that they would not be capable of being a good parent. As Woollett and Marshall (2000, p. 313) note, 'motherhood is construed as problematic for those women who do not bring up children in the "right" circumstances at the "right" time', and being young is one of the circumstances which results in being excluded from the category of good mother. Australian (Mulherin and Johnstone 2015) and Canadian (Whitley and Kirmayer 2008) research suggests that mothers in their early twenties feel as stigmatised as teenagers due to being relatively young, particularly with the average age of mothers reaching 30 in both countries (as it is in the UK). However, like the young women in the studies discussed above, the young parents and parents-to-be here felt that despite others' perceptions, their age was irrelevant:

> I don't like the way people see young parents, just because of my age doesn't mean I'm not perfectly capable taking care of my own child. (Becky)

Older mothers also discussed the same perceptions. Paula, who had become a mother at 16, and whose daughter was pregnant aged 15, had experienced 'being talked down to' herself, and had also supported her niece (mother at age 19) and her daughter-in-law (mother at age 18) when they had felt unsupported and criticised by health care professionals:

> They think just because you are a young mum you don't know nothing and you are talked down to.

Hirst et al. (2006) also found that the stigma of being a young parent was something that was common to the different generations in their study. However, both younger and older parents felt that age was irrelevant in terms of ability to be a good parent, and in many cases the young people had a great deal of experience of looking after younger relatives. Becky, for example, quoted above, had spent her early teens looking after her four younger siblings to try to keep them out of care because their mother had a drug problem. In other cases, families were often very close geographically as well as being involved in each other's lives. As in Mitchell and Green's (2002) study and going even further back, Young and Willmot (1962), seeing female relatives daily, or at least several times a week, was normal, as was helping to look after other small children in the family.

After emphasising that anyone could be a good or a bad parent regardless of age, the young parents then went on to describe the advantages of being young, the obvious one being having more energy. In some cases they also felt that younger parents coped better with a baby, because parenthood could come as a shock to older people who had had a career:

> Parents that are older, that have had their career and then they get a baby, and they think 'I'll be able to do this because my life's worked out', and it just throws them out, and I think because you are young, you just get on with it, don't you? It doesn't like faze you as much. (Faye)

They were also aware of the discourse about putting careers first and the dangers of 'leaving it too late':

> They put their career first, and by the time they think 'I'm sorted, I want kids' it's too late sort of thing, they've picked career over a family. (Zara)

Being labelled in a negative way was something that the participants were aware of both as the wider context for their experience, in that they knew the commonly held assumptions about teenage parents, but also for many of them it was something they had experienced face to face through comments overheard on the bus or in the street, or in several instances, remarks made directly to them. Megan suggested that while she had experienced some people questioning her abilities as a young mother, it was due to nosiness, and not that they made her feel judged. She felt that people in her community were mainly accepting of teenage parents:

> I think you get the odd one or two people which are like 'how's she going to cope, she's so young', this and that, and you always get the odd one or two, or they come on to you and they're like 'how you doing?', you know, trying to nose, I reckon. But you do get, there's some people which are like, do you know, 'I reckon you lot are brilliant parents, I reckon you lot are better than me when I was older than you having kids'. That's what I reckon, you get the odd one or two, but there's a good community ... I never had people like judging me. But I'm just like, I'm just me, I don't care what other people think as long as I know that my kids are well looked after, I don't care what anyone else thinks.

Media coverage was felt to be pervasive and influential, resulting in everyone being 'tarred with the same brush' (Nikki). It was felt that negative stereotypes were common on television and in newspapers:

> Jamie   They all have their typical stereotypes though and they don't take into account everybody's individual situation so they look at BBC News and stuff, see stuff on the news, and then they suddenly think that—
>
> Naomi   —that's how everyone is. There's never anything good [in the papers], I think that's what portrays us as bad people, bad parents.

Yet while they were very aware that they were being labelled and stigmatised, with people making assumptions not only about their ability as parents but also about the rest of their life, they were conscious that this was a stereotype and that they operated within a moral discourse of teenage parenting being about low aspirations and life on benefits:

> When you do talk about teenage parents, you do think stereotypical on the dole, you know, not having any aspirations in life but I think that's just like saying black people can dance, you know? (everyone laughs) (Sharon)

However, as with the respondents in Clarke's study, 'there was no evidence of a culture of dependency on benefits' (2013, p. 12), and no resemblance in either study to the persistent portrayals of young women getting pregnant deliberately in order to access benefits and housing. They may need benefits, but this is regarded as a temporary measure. This is in part because, as in the studies discussed by Duncan (2007), parenthood had made many of them more driven and more determined to succeed, either by going back to an education that had been interrupted by pregnancy, or by beginning to pursue training and qualifications because they had responsibilities:

> I think it makes you want to prove that you can still do it. For me anyway, when I got pregnant people said to me 'you're going to be on benefits all your life, you may as well forget about what you want to do'. I don't see why having a child means that I have to give up on what I wanted to do in the first place, and it just makes me more motivated to finish things, go back to college and get a job. (Jenny)

In contrast to always being regarded negatively, Jamie said that he felt he was respected sometimes because he countered the stereotypes of feckless fathers:

> I think I get a lot more respect off people because, like, I think the men have got a reputation of just getting someone pregnant and then bunking, so because I've stuck by them both, I think I get a lot of positive comments by trying to support them rather than just bailing.

The staff focus group in Norland discussed the stigma attached to young parents, and like Jamie, felt that young fathers would receive very different reactions to young mothers:

> If you then looked at stigma attached to young dads, a young dad with a baby and a pram would be 'oh isn't he wonderful, what a good dad!' Whereas a young mum with a baby would be 'oh God!' So even within young parents, male and female, there's a different kind of stigma. (Carol)

Katy had been interviewed by the local paper shortly before being interviewed for the study, as an example of a successful young mum:

> I mean I've done a case study which was in the [local paper] and things like that and I've done a few interviews and a speech about being a teen parent but nobody has ever sort of said to me 'I think that's wrong'.

However, despite saying here that no-one had criticised her for being a young parent, she then went on to give examples of people commenting behind her back on the bus:

> You get it a lot from people when you're sat on the bus, like when I'm sat there with Josh and you get younger girls going 'aww' and then he'll have a paddy and they're like 'oh God, can't control a kiddie,' it's like 'yeah, you're 15, you come and do it, you come and do it if you think you can do it'.

Jamie and Katy, along with Megan, were in the minority in terms of having received a positive reaction to being a young parent. Overwhelmingly, the young parents in this generation and the older generations had experienced negative reactions from strangers, as indeed at times had Jamie, Katy and Megan. This led them all to expect surveillance and judgement from strangers in the wider community.

Surveillance and Judgement

The consequence of being labelled and stigmatised as a young parent was that many of them felt that they were being watched, being given funny or nasty looks, being whispered about on the bus, and being judged all the time, for what they were wearing, how they behaved, and how their children behaved. Again, this watching and judging is linked to the stereotype of teen/bad parent:

> I think there's more of a stereotype now ... I always feel like somcone is judging you. (Dave)

In this exchange in a focus group, Zara mentions her fear of going out if her daughter had a scratch or a bruise, in case 'someone at the bus stop' saw her and reported her to Social Services; Jenny suggests that younger and older parents are regarded differently in this situation:

Zara   It's like the other week, she got scratched by the cat, and I know people are thinking 'what's that?', thinking 'well, she's done that', sort of thing, like at the minute she's got a bruise on her face and I'm expecting people to think I've done it to her.

Jenny If you were older, people would say kids hurt themselves and stuff but because you are young, they always seem to assume that you've made a mistake or, do you know … Well, I don't know whether people do actually assume this but this is how we feel.

Jenny's acknowledgement here that she doesn't actually know if people are making assumptions about her, but she thinks that they are, was a common feeling. The young parents become hyperaware of looks and whispers, as Wenham (2015) found, to the extent that in some cases, the fear of judgement overrides experience. Zara's fear of someone at the bus stop reporting her to Social Services contrasts with what has actually happened at the bus stop, which is next to sheltered accommodation for older people:

> I go to the bus stop at the top, by the roundabout, and there's like an old people's home. And they all come out and talk to me at the bus stop while they are waiting for the bus, and they'll say 'aww, isn't she cute?' and stuff.

Despite her positive experiences with older people complimenting her on her baby, she is fearful of potential negative experiences that have not yet happened. Zara also chose not to attend a local playgroup, in case there were older mothers there who might judge her for being young; Nikki had attended a playgroup with older mothers and had stopped attending because no-one would speak to her. Vincent and Thomson (2013) found that the pressure to prove themselves as mothers meant young mothers avoided places where they felt others might look down on them, and this certainly seems to be the case here. These feelings of constant judgement and fear of others led to many of the young parents feeling very defensive about their abilities, and as if they have to prove themselves to people such as health visitors. In turn this led to feelings of stress and tension. Whitley and Kirmayer (2008) suggested that the women in their study, who were mothers in their early twenties, experienced the same level of stigmatisation as teenage mothers, with 'deleterious effects' on their health, particularly mental health, as a consequence. It seems reasonable to suggest that the constant defensiveness and pressure to prove that they did not conform to negative stereotypes felt by participants in this study could have an impact on their mental health.

Whereas Yardley found that the negative effects of stigma were less for women where young motherhood was not unusual in their families, and as a result were 'insulated from negative criticism' (2008, p. 681) this did not appear to be the case in this study. All the women here come from a background where young motherhood is part of their family history, but they still reported feeling stigmatised and judged, and in many cases had experienced negative criticism from outside the family. Within the family, they worked to counter this by demonstrating either that the young mother had the experience to be a good mother through having cared for babies and young children (as was the case with Debbie and Haley), or that they would learn within a supportive home (as was the case with Zara and her mother Janet). However, despite this family work, the negative feeling of being labelled and judged persisted.

Parenthood as a Turning Point

Studies from the UK and the USA show that motherhood is often positive for young women despite the stigma attached to it (Duncan 2007), and that it can be a turning point (Clarke 2013). In particular, becoming a mother can act as an incentive for young women to complete their education in order to get a better job as they now have a baby to provide for (SmithBattle 2007b; Vincent and Thomson 2010; Leese 2014).

Austerberry and Wiggins (2007) caution against the emphasis on returning to education, particularly as it was promoted by Sure Start Plus, as the pressure to return to school or college works for those young mothers who wanted to continue their education but not for those who were disengaged with schooling before they were pregnant. However, a number of studies show that even those who are disengaged are motivated towards education once they become a mother, although clearly this does not apply to everyone. Not doing well with academic subjects or being unhappy at school was a common feature of the life stories the young women told, as Megan explained earlier.

Whilst Katy is an example of someone who was highly motivated to obtain qualifications, having previously drifted between courses she did not really like at school as well as at college, both Amy (17) and Sarah (15) had been moved out of mainstream schooling and into pupil referral units. Amy said she found school boring, and acknowledged that her attitude had been poor. For Sarah, not only had she been moved out of school because, as her mother Paula said, she was 'having trouble at school before she became pregnant', she had also been told she could no longer attend the unit 'because of health and safety'. Amy said that she had applied to go to college, but later said she had not decided whether she wanted to do hairdressing or cooking. Although Sarah said she would think about going to college later, in the interview her mother seemed much keener on her getting some qualifications that Sarah did.

Where young women do want to continue at school while pregnant, and return once their baby is born, evidence from the UK (Vincent and Thomson 2010) and the USA (SmithBattle 2007b) suggests that successful continuation and return is very heavily contingent on supportive teachers and school authorities. In some cases, this might mean moving to a specialised unit; Haley had been at school when she found out she was pregnant but had been unable to continue attending due to sickness:

> I was at sixth form, and I was about two months into it, and I found out I was pregnant. I left because I had to be there all the time, I couldn't handle it because I was real badly.

As a result of her poor attendance record, and other bad experiences, she had decided to leave school. However, she did not want to give up her education. Her mother, Tina, had been one of the first girls to attend a new 'schoolgirl mums' unit when she was a pregnant teenager, so Haley asked her to help get a place at the now well-established unit:

> I said to my mam I didn't want to sit at home all the time and just lounge about, so I got my mam to talk to [head teacher] for me.

For others, it could be a turning point in terms of being an incentive to return to education or training, and find meaningful employment; Katy had undertaken training and was working as a trainee youth advisor:

> If I hadn't had Josh I wouldn't have gone on any of my courses, I wouldn't have got in at anywhere because I didn't know what I wanted to do and I'd left it too late and I'd've ended up just being on dole probably and ending up with jobs that I don't like, whereas now I'm teaching and I get to support people doing things, you know going through things that I've been through and, you know, I have like a lot of people around me now who are proud of me for what I have done, and if I hadn't have done that, I'd have ended up just working in my dad's shop in the end because he would have had enough of me, he'd have just said 'get to work' and that'll be it … my life would be crap to be fair (laughs).

Most of those who had been at school or college were keen to return to their education, although for those at school that meant going to college instead, as school attendance could be challenging, both in terms of workload and in terms of reactions from other pupils. As we saw in Chapter 4, Naomi, who seemed to have had a particularly bad experience, had suffered bullying from other pupils because she was pregnant, which led to her dropping out of sixth form. Her younger sister had also become caught up in the bullying:

> My little sister goes to the school I went to, and I went to the sixth form at that school, and one girl said to her 'oh, is your sister pregnant?' and she said 'yeah' and they said 'oh, she's a right slag' to my sister, my little sister who's 14 at the time.

At the time of first interviewing her, Naomi was at home with her son, aged four months. By the time of the second interview four months later, she had started a college course, although she had not been able to continue her plans to become a teacher:

> I didn't want to drop out completely so I just changed courses to a two-day course on hairdressing, which turns out I do want to carry on with that now, just a backup in case, because I just didn't want to drop out, do you know what I mean? But I did want to be an English specialist teacher.

Because of discrimination, bullying, or other negative experiences, many young women who become pregnant while still at school experience damage to their education which has long-lasting consequences. Vincent and Thomson highlight that for many of these young women, who take college courses in beauty, hairdressing or social and child care, their future earnings potential and employment security is damaged, and therefore 'the consequences of their school experiences are thus more than simply social exclusion but are also economic and political' (Vincent and Thomson 2010, p. 382).

The young parents countered the problematic nature of teenage parenting by acknowledging that it was perceived as a problem and in a negative light, then explaining why it was not so for them:

> The fact that I knew it wasn't the end of the world to have a baby at this age which it isn't, I'm doing better than I was before, I'm happier now. People make out your life is over once you have a baby if you're young because you won't get to go out as much. The way I see it, I'll get to go out now and again because my mam and dad will have him now and again, and I get to come home to a baby and they get to go home to a hangover or whatever, so it doesn't bother me really. I'm just more sensible in myself … I never used to be scared, like if we went out I'd go 'yeah let's do that, let's do that' but now I think maybe I shouldn't. I'm in a lot less danger than I used to be. (Haley)

Not only is it not the end of the world, having a baby brings positive changes, for Haley being more sensible, for others having a new direction, more confidence, and a sense of accomplishment.

Conclusions

Despite almost all the pregnancies being unintended, motherhood was embraced by all the young women in the study, as it had been embraced in turn by the older generations. Not all the fathers had been so enthusiastic, and in some cases young men who had encouraged their girlfriends to get pregnant or to keep the baby had not remained in the relationship, and in a few cases had not had anything to do with their child either. Although the young parents discussed some of the challenges and difficulties of their new role, such as tiredness, lack of money, being cut off from old friends and social lives, and being judged by others around them, they also talked about the enjoyment they got from being a parent, saying they 'wouldn't change it for the world'.

In some cases, becoming a parent had acted as a turning point, whereby those who had not been in education or had been uncertain about their future had found a new determination and direction now that they had someone to care for. They were keen to demonstrate that they were good parents, and that they were taking on the responsibility knowingly and willingly. Like the parents in Hirst et al.'s (2006) study, having children gave a sense of purpose, and putting the child first was both a requirement of being a good parent, and proof, if they did it, that someone was good. For those who had been in work or in education, a baby provided a further spur to succeed, particularly for the young fathers who were actively taking on a breadwinner role.

The participants in the study are well aware of the discourses around teenage pregnancy and parenthood, and are aware of their position in a stigmatised group about whom value judgements are made, by politicians, the media, and people around them, in their communities, their schools, and on the streets. However, they were all very clear about distinguishing themselves from this discourse by constructing an identity as a good mother (McDermott and Graham 2005; Romagnoli and Wall 2012), what Kirkman et al. (2001) call a 'consoling plot'. All the participants rejected the notion of becoming pregnant in order to have a life on benefits, and those on benefits expressed a strong desire to get out of the benefit system and support themselves as soon as this was practical.

It is clear that the three key dimensions to stigma (Scambler and Hopkins 1986; Scambler and Paoli 2008) are operating in the lives of the young people in this study. Enacted stigma, in the form of being seen as imperfect, or deviant, exists both indirectly, in the stories in the media about young parents, and directly, in the looks and comments made to and about them. As a response, they experience felt stigma, in that they know they are supposed to feel shame; however, they resist a shamed identity very strongly, and reject the negative stereotypes which would label them as bad parents, and as Naomi said, 'bad people'. In this sense, they are displaying project stigma, in terms of their strategies of resistance to the stigmatised identity of 'teen parent'. These strategies include ensuring that they and their babies are well dressed and look cared for, but also sometimes involve avoiding settings where they might feel judged. Public stigma (Scambler 2004, 2009), in the form of prejudices arising from the adoption of stereotypes by the general population, means that they are constantly aware of how they might be judged, so they need to be prepared for it at all times. They also distance themselves from stigma by agreeing that the stereotypical 'bad parent' exists, but they are not, as they can demonstrate that they are good. In doing this, they are operating what Kingfisher calls a 'bad people exist but I'm not one of them' discourse (1996, p. 56), and creating a mental divide between good selves and bad others (Mitchell and Green 2002) that is protective.

The young parents have a further protection from enacted and public stigma in that they are part of families who have value systems where young motherhood is accepted (Yardley 2008), and creating the next generation is worthy and welcomed. The next chapter looks at how the wider family responds to the new baby, and in what ways these responses have altered or remained the same across the generations.

References

Austerberry, H., & Wiggins, M. (2007). Taking a pro-choice perspective on promoting inclusion of teenage mothers: Lessons from an evaluation of the Sure Start Plus programme. *Critical Public Health, 17*(1), 3–15.

Breheny, M., & Stephens, C. (2007). Individual responsibility and social constraint: The construction of adolescent motherhood in social scientific research. *Culture, Health & Sexuality, 9*(4), 333–346.

Brown, S., & Guthrie, K. (2010). Why don't teenagers use contraception? A qualitative interview study. *European Journal of Contraception and Reproductive Health Care, 15*, 197–204.

Clarke, J. (2013). It's not all doom and gloom for teenage mothers – Exploring the factors that contribute to positive outcomes. *International Journal of Adolescence and Youth.* doi:10.1080/02673843.2013.804424.

Duncan, S. (2007). What's the problem with teenage parents? And what's the problem with policy? *Critical Social Policy, 27*(3), 307–334.

Graham, H., & McDermott, E. (2006). Qualitative research and the evidence base of policy: Insights from studies of teenage mothers in the UK. *Journal of Social Policy, 35*(1), 21–37.

Hansen, K., Hawkes, D., & Joshi, H. (2009). The timing of motherhood, mothers' employment and child outcomes. In J. Stillwell, E. Coast, & D. Kneale (Eds.), *Fertility, living arrangements, care and mobility. Understanding population trends and processes, Vol. 1*. London: Springer.

Hirst, J., Formby, E., & Owen, J. (2006). *Pathways into parenthood: Reflections from three generations of teenage mothers and fathers*. Sheffield: Sheffield Hallam University, Sheffield Health and Social Research Consortium.

Jewell, D., Tacchi, J., & Donovan, J. (2000). Teenage pregnancy: Whose problem is it? *Family Practice, 17*(6), 522–528.

Kingfisher, C. P. (1996). *Women in the American welfare trap*. Philadelphia, PA: University of Pennsylvania Press.

Kirkman, M., Harrison, M., Hillier, L., & Pyett, P. (2001). 'I know I'm doing a good job': Canonical and autobiographical narratives of teenage mothers. *Culture, Health and Sexuality, 3*(3), 279–294.

Leese, M. (2014). The 'bumpy road' to becoming: Capturing the stories that teenage mothers told about their journey into motherhood. *Child and Family Social Work.* doi:10.1111/cfs.12169.

Maruna, S. (2001). *Making good: How ex-convicts reform and rebuild their lives*. Washington, DC: American Psychological Association.

McDermott, E., & Graham, H. (2005). Resilient young mothering: Social inequalities, late modernity and the 'problem' of 'teenage' motherhood. *Journal of Youth Studies, 8*(1), 59–79.

Mitchell, W., & Green, E. (2002). 'I don't know what I'd do without our Mam' motherhood, identity and support networks. *The Sociological Review, 50*, 1–22.

Mollborn, S., & Jacobs, J. (2015). 'I'll be there for you': Teen parents' co-parenting relationships. *Journal of Marriage and Family, 77*(2), 373–387.

Moorhead, J. (2015). We're glad we chose to be mothers in our teens. *The Guardian.* Retrieved September 30, 2015, from http://www.theguardian.com/lifeandstyle/2015/jan/10/were-glad-we-chose-to-be-mothers-in-our-teens

Mulherin, K., & Johnstone, M. (2015). Qualitative accounts of teenage and emerging adult women adjusting to motherhood. *Journal of Reproductive and Infant Psychology, 33*(4), 388–401.

Phoenix, A. (1991). *Young mothers*. Cambridge: Polity Press.

Rolfe, A. (2008). 'You've got to grow up when you've got a kid': Marginalized young women's accounts of motherhood. *Journal of Community and Applied Social Psychology, 18*, 299–314.

Romagnoli, A., & Wall, G. (2012). 'I know I'm a good mom': Young, low income mothers' experiences with risk perception, intensive parenting ideology and parenting education programmes. *Health, Risk and Society, 14*(3), 273–289.

Scambler, G. (2004). Reframing stigma: Felt and enacted stigma and challenges to the sociology of chronic and disabling conditions. *Social Theory and Health, 2*, 29–46.

Scambler, G. (2009). Health-related stigma. *Sociology of Health and Illness, 31*, 441–455.

Scambler, G., & Hopkins, A. (1986). Being epileptic: Coming to terms with stigma. *Sociology of Health and Illness, 8*, 26–43.

Scambler, G., & Paoli, F. (2008). Health work, female sex workers and HIV/AIDS: Global and local dimensions of stigma and deviance as barriers to effective interventions. *Social Science and Medicine, 66*(8), 1848–1862.

Shibutani, T. (1955). Reference groups as perspectives. *American Journal of Sociology, 60*(6), 562–569.

Smith, S., & Ratcliffe, A. (2009). Women's education and childbearing: A growing divide. In J. Stillwell, E. Coast, & D. Kneale (Eds.), *Fertility, living arrangements, care and mobility. Understanding population trends and processes, vol. 1*. London: Springer.

SmithBattle, L. (2007a). Legacies of advantage and disadvantage: The case of teen mothers. *Public Health Nursing, 24*(5), 409–420.

SmithBattle, L. (2007b). 'I wanna have a good future': Teen mothers' rise in educational aspirations, competing demands and limited school support. *Youth and Society, 38*(3), 348–371.

Vincent, K., & Thomson, P. (2010). 'Slappers like you don't belong in this school': The educational inclusion/exclusion of pregnant schoolgirls. *International Journal of Inclusive Education, 14*(4), 371–385.

Vincent, K., & Thomson, P. (2013). 'Your age don't determine whether you're a good mum': Reframing the discourse of deviance ascribed to teenage mothers. *Social Alternatives, 32*(2), 6–12.

Wenham, A. (2015). 'I know I'm a good mum – No one can tell me different': Young mothers negotiating a stigmatised identity through time. *Families, Relationships and Societies*, doi:10.1332/204674315X14193466354732

Whitley, R., & Kirmayer, L. J. (2008). Perceived stigmatisation of young mothers: An exploratory study of psychological and social experience. *Social Science and Medicine, 66*, 339–348.

Woollett, A., & Marshall, H. (2000). Motherhood and mothering. In J. Ussher (Ed.), *Women's health: Contemporary international perspectives*. Leicester: British Psychological Society.

Yardley, E. (2008). Teenage mothers' experiences of stigma. *Journal of Youth Studies, 11*(6), 671–684.

Young, M., & Willmot, P. (1962). *Family and kinship in East London*. Harmondsworth: Penguin.

6

'It's Bringing New Life in': The Baby and the Wider Family

This chapter describes the family settings in which the young people live, and considers how the teenage parents and their babies fit into the wider family, including grandparents and other relatives. It also considers how the participants in the study constructed the idea of family, based on Morgan's concept of family practices, whereby families are sets of activities rather than structures or groups to which individual members belong. As Finch (2007) argues, citing Morgan, family is an aspect of social life rather than an institution, representing 'a quality rather than a thing' (Morgan 1996, p. 186). In this chapter I concentrate largely on the four families who took part in the study where more than one generation was interviewed, although I also draw on the other interviews and focus groups where participants talked about their families. In this way it is possible to draw out the intergenerational relationships, and the experiences of teenage parenting across the generations.

Policy approaches to family tend to take a specific and somewhat narrow view of what constitutes a family, 'which reflects more an ideological construction than a reflection of lived experiences' (Morgan 2013, p. 50) and is based on the 'standard North American family' (Smith 1993,

© The Editor(s) (if applicable) and The Author(s) 2016

S. Brown, *Teenage Pregnancy, Parenting and Intergenerational Relations,*
DOI 10.1057/978-1-137-49539-6_6

cited in Morgan 2013). The conventional, or traditional, notion of the nuclear family with two heterosexual parents and their children forming a household does not reflect modern lived experience of single parenting, step-parenting and blended families, or gay couples and their children; although statistics indicate that there were 12.5 million married couple families in the UK in 2014 (out of 18.6 million families), cohabiting couple families were the fastest growing family type and there were two million lone parent families, whilst 28 per cent of households contained only one person, and the fastest growing household type recently has been households containing two or more families (ONS 2015). As Finch (2007) points out, and the data indicate, a family does not equate to a household. However in policy terms, and in the way many politicians approach talking about families, there is an assumption that 'household' and 'nuclear family' overlap.

Policy specifically regarding teenage pregnancy and parenting also positions teenage parenting as a route to social exclusion, as discussed earlier. Comparing the lived experiences of the families in this study with the 'wider cultural and political view of teenage motherhood that is profoundly negative' (Macvarish 2010, p. 319) challenges this overwhelming negativity. As Macvarish points out, along with Thomson (2000) and Lee et al. (2004), there is a disjuncture between the way families talk about the new baby and how he or she fits in to patterns of regenerating the family, and the way politicians and policymakers talk about teenage parents and their children. This chapter questions the emphasis on social exclusion as a consequence of teenage parenting that is usually seen in policy approaches, and counters the impression often given that teenage parents are socially isolated and somehow 'apart' from society.

Using Morgan's concept of family practices as a lens through which to view classic texts such as Young and Wilmott's *Family and Kinship in East London* (1962) and Cornwell's *Hard earned lives; accounts of health and illness from East London* (1984), caring was a practice undertaken vertically across three, sometimes four, generations, and horizontally between siblings and cousins, whereby grandmothers would, for example, care for their grandchildren and women would care for their sisters' and cousins' children. The case studies I discuss in this chapter illustrate a continuation of those family practices in ways that have not changed dramatically for many families in the 50-plus years since the publication of *Family and Kinship in East London*. I begin by introducing each family.

The Baker Family

The matriarch of the Baker family, Cathy, had five children, three girls and two boys, the first being born when Cathy was 18. Paula, the second daughter, was interviewed for this study as was her daughter, Sarah. All three of Cathy's daughters had their first children when they were teenagers, Paula's older sister having hers when she was 15, and Paula having Sarah's older brother Luke when she was 17 and Sarah when she was 19. Some of Cathy's grandchildren have also had children in their teens, so at age 58, Cathy has five children, eight grandchildren and five great-grandchildren (including Sarah's as yet unborn baby). Cathy was married before her first daughter was born, but is now divorced.

Paula's son Luke had twins with his girlfriend when he was 16 and she was 18; they live together and he worked full-time, although shortly after the interview with Paula, he was made redundant and he and his family moved in with Paula, who also has a younger son (aged 11) at home as well as Sarah. Paula has been together with her partner since she was 16 and he was 19; they moved in together when Paula was 17 and pregnant, having been asked to leave home by her father. They have never married. He works full-time.

Sarah got pregnant when she was 15, and will be 16 when her baby is born. Her boyfriend is 20 and already has one child, with whom he has contact. They plan to move in together once the baby is born.

The Fox Family

Janet Fox, age 41, left home at 16 to move in with her boyfriend; her parents had divorced when she was six, and she spent the next few years living with her mother, younger sister and step-father, then living with her father, and then moving in with her boyfriend. Her first son was born when she was 17, but when she was pregnant with her second son at the age of 18, she left her home due to her partner's violence. She was homeless for a while, and moved between her father's flat and friends' homes before marrying a new partner and having Zara when she was 22. Her marriage broke down because her husband was violent towards both Janet and Zara. Zara had her daughter, Ellie, when she was 19. Ellie's father is not involved with her; Zara has not seen him since before Ellie was born. Janet, her new partner (referred to as 'my stepdad' by Zara), Zara and the baby live together. Janet's older son has two small children, a daughter, aged six, born when he was 19 and who now lives with him, and a son, aged four, who lives with his mother. He is no longer in a relationship with either of the mothers of his children. Janet regularly cares for his daughter.

The Smith Family

Tina Smith is 35, and has three daughters and one son. She described a very troubled childhood, characterised by abuse, violence, truanting from school, and running away from home. She had her first daughter when she was 14, and described how she had featured in a national newspaper as a 'gymslip mum'. When she left hospital with her first baby, she was taken in by a family friend. Tina and the friend's son, Kevin, began their relationship when she was 16, and together they have three children, two daughters and a son, and are married. Kevin teaches at a local college, and at the time of the interviews was busy finishing the building of a large kitchen/dining room extension to their house. All three of Tina's daughters have had children as teenagers; Haley, the youngest, was 16 when she had her son Riley. Riley's father is not involved with the baby, indeed he has denied paternity. Haley and Riley live with Tina and Kevin, and her younger brother.

The Jones Family

Sheila Jones, aged 41, has three children, two sons in their twenties and Debbie, aged 17. Debbie's baby will be Sheila's first grandchild. Sheila was 15 when her oldest son was born; she lived at home with her mother and her son until the baby was two. She met Phil, they settled down together, and had two children. All three children live at home. Phil works full-time, and Sheila has two part-time jobs. Her mother Eileen was 24 when Sheila was born, becoming a grandmother at 39 when Sheila had her first baby. She also works part-time in a care home. Eileen's sister Mary, aged 72, had her first child when she was 17, and just married to her first and only boyfriend, who was in the army. Mary lived with his mother until her husband came out of the army and they could set up home together with their baby son. They had another three children. Eileen and Mary have five brothers and sisters. Eileen, Mary, Sheila and Sheila's two sisters all live within a short walking distance of each other, and see each other several times a week. Eileen has two great-grandchildren (Debbie's cousin's twins) who she looks after regularly, often with Debbie's help.

The Jones family were interviewed as a group. Sheila, her mother Eileen ('say I'm in my early sixties'), and Eileen's sister Mary (72) took part along with Debbie. Debbie's father Phil was also at home, and joined the discussion part way through.

The Young People

Several interviews took place with young people where it was not possible to speak to other members of their families. I relied on a snowball approach, where I asked the initial interviewee to ask their parents and/or partners whether they would also like to take part. This worked once, when Naomi was interviewed for the second time with her partner Jamie. Boyfriends were often described as 'not very talkative', not worth asking because he was shy, or 'you won't get much out of him', so it may be the case that the initial participant decided not to pass the invitation on. In cases of estrangement, either from partner or parent, clearly there was not going to be an opportunity for an invitation to be passed on. However, despite the unavailability of other family members for interviews, several young people talked at length about their families of upbringing, and their thoughts and feelings about their new family, and these individuals will also feature in this chapter. In particular, Katy, Naomi and Jamie had contrasting family backgrounds and different living arrangements at the time of the interviews; they had clear ideas about the meaning of family for them, and these are described here.

Katy

Katy had her son Josh when she was 17 and Josh's father Pete was 19; they had been together since she was 15, but had split up at the time of Katie's interviews (we met twice). Pete has subsequently had another son, but is no longer with the mother of that child, and has a new girlfriend. He cares for Josh on a regular basis, having him to stay overnight twice a week. He also sees his new son, Josh's half-brother. Katy was born when her mother was 18 years old. Her parents divorced when she was very young; her father remarried when Katy was three, and she has a good relationship with her stepmother. Her mother has had several relationships, and has twins aged four. Katy ran away from home to be with Pete when she found out she was pregnant (interestingly she chooses to talk about running away, rather than saying she moved in with her partner), and was estranged from both parents for most of her pregnancy. Now, though, she and Josh see her father regularly and Josh is close to his grandfather. Katy was supported by her grandmother during her pregnancy, but her grandmother died shortly after Josh was born. Katy has her own house where she lives with Josh; she is on an apprenticeship and completing national vocational qualifications (NVQs).

Naomi and Jamie

Naomi and Jamie are 17 and 18 respectively, and live together with their son Jordan. They plan to get married in a year or two. Naomi is the third of four girls in her family; her mother had Naomi's oldest sister when she was 19. Neither of Naomi's older sisters have children. Her younger sister is 14 and still at school. Jamie has two brothers, neither of whom have children, so Jordan is the first grandchild for both sets of grandparents. Naomi and Jamie's parents acted as guarantors for the privately rented house they live in. Naomi had just completed her GCSEs when she found out she was pregnant; she had planned to carry on with A levels and had hoped to go to university (she was unusual amongst the young women to have this ambition) but has decided that is no longer possible, and by the time of her second interview had started a part-time hairdressing course. Jamie is at college doing A levels, and intends to go to university, which was his plan before he and Naomi had Jordan and settled down together.

Multigenerational Experiences

Most of the literature about multigenerational experiences of family life, where three generations live together in the same household, is American, and much of that is focussed on research with African American families, particularly those where one family member is a teenage parent. Burton (1990), for example, looked at a small African American community and found that poor families had 'accelerated timetables' of progression through family life, with parenthood in the teens and grandparenthood in the thirties, in contrast to what she calls American middle-class norms. Hunter (1997) suggests that the social and cultural structures of African American families mean that the role of grandparents and the focus on multigenerational family arrangements are more significant than marriage. In this sense, having an involved grandmother is a well-established family strategy. Chase-Lansdale et al. (1994) found that for the youngest teenage mothers, living with their mother was beneficial for the baby, but this was not the case for older teens. The paper is imprecise in terms of what they regard as younger and older teens, but in the light of other research it would be unsurprising to find that a 14-year-old mother needed more support from her mother than a 19-year-old would. Dunifon and Kowaleski-Jones (2007) suggested that poorer outcomes (for the children) in some studies where a grandmother and mother co-resided could be due to the mother needing support which meant she lived with the grandmother, rather than the living arrangement per se. Similarly, Goodman (2007) found that some three-generation families form because of the immaturity of the young mother, although evidence about outcomes was mixed. What she called connected families, who communicated well and where the grandparent respected the autonomy of the parent, did well; disconnected families did less well, but this may well have been because they had other problems such as substance abuse. Overall, she found that three-generation families did better than skipped generation ones, that is, families where the grandparent raised the baby without the input of the parent. In their longitudinal study of single parents in multigenerational families, Deleire and Kalil (2002) suggested that young mothers on a low income may benefit from living in a multi-generational household, particularly in terms of developmental outcomes for their children. This, they argue, could be due to the resources pro-vided by grandparents that mitigate the effects of poverty. Grandparents also influence the development of a young mother's parenting skills when they live together in a multigenerational household (SmithBattle 2006).

None of the families who took part in my study were skipped genera-tion families, and most were three-generation, at least in the early part of the baby's life. We have already heard how many of the mothers and fathers reacted to their daughters' pregnancies; the rest of this chapter discusses how the families worked, across the generations, focussing on the older members: the mothers, fathers and grandmothers of the young parents.

Hoping for Better

One of the common responses from the parents and grandparents of the teenagers who were pregnant was that they had wanted better for their daughters, which was why news of the pregnancies had initially resulted in disappointment:

> I was upset at first because I wanted a bit more for her, but now we've got used to it. (Eileen, Debbie's grandmother)
> I wanted better for them but I've always told them that. I haven't said 'oh, it's a good thing, it's ok', I've told them, you know, tried to give them good advice. (Paula, Sarah's mother)

What comprises 'better' was rarely articulated in detail, and seems to rest on an unspoken assumption that most parents will hope that their chil-dren have better lives than they have had. Paula mentions money and jobs:

> I'm not saying having children is wrong, I'm not saying that. I just wanted things to be a little bit different for my own, you know, not to struggle and to have money behind them and have jobs.

Here, as discussed earlier, she encapsulates the dilemma faced by the mothers of pregnant teenagers who had been teenage mothers themselves, of how to articulate their wish for their children to wait to become parents without making it sound as if they regretted having had those children. Mostly, the wish was that they had waited until they had some financial security. In Paula's case she and her partner had set up home together when they were teenagers, and he had always had a job:

> Sarah's dad's always worked, so he said 'I'll get the work and you, if that's what you want, you look after the children.'

The wish for 'something better' seems to revolve around financial security within relatively proscribed limits; it is about having a job, or finishing a college course so that the young parent can get a job later, rather than wanting their child to have gone to university, to move away, or to have a career. None of the parents talked about university or described the pregnancy in terms of a thwarted career, which raises a number of questions about aspirations and expectations.

By saying that 'we wanted better', the parents seemed to be saying that they wanted their children to have higher aspirations, but in fact what they want their children to aspire to is not a university degree and a high-flying career, it is having a job, and probably not that dissimilar a job to themselves. Debbie, for example, was at college doing a course in childcare when she found out she was pregnant; her mother Sheila has one job in a care home and another job as a 'dinner lady' in a nearby primary school, and Sheila's mother Eileen also has a part-time job in a care home. Debbie will, in due course, probably get a job in care work, although with children rather than with elderly people. In this sense, Sheila and Eileen do not want Debbie to have that different a life to the ones they lead, but they wish she had waited until she had finished her training before she had her baby.

Although two studies from New Zealand (Boden et al. 2008; Gibb et al. 2014) found a lasting impact on economic outcomes for teenage parents compared to non-parents, most research which has attempted to evaluate the impact on life chances of pregnancy and motherhood at a young age suggests that becoming a parent as a teenager did not have a radical impact on teenagers' life paths and socio-economic status (Geronimus and Korenman 1992, 1993; Hotz et al. 1996; Furstenberg 2007; Lawlor et al. 2011). Despite this, parents still wish for better for their children, seemingly unaware that according to much of the research, early parenthood makes little difference to long-term outcomes. This can possibly be explained by a disconnection between what people know about the wider context, and what they hope for individually; they may know that very few people from their locality have radically different lives to their parents, but they hope that their children will have better lives than they have had. By examining the idea of 'better', in the way that Paula and Sheila talked about it, we see that for many people it means small increments—having a job, having a little more financial security—not radical difference.

Models of Motherhood

Young women can take one of two approaches to how they 'do' parenting and raise their child: either modelling themselves on their own mother, or making their own version of motherhood based on being not like their mother. The longitudinal study carried out by SmithBattle (1996, 1997, 2000, 2006) shows how care-giving legacies and family practices influenced the way teenage mothers chose to be a parent. Those with positive experiences from childhood imitated the way their parents had cared for them, whereas those with negative experiences attempted to develop more positive parenting styles in opposition to the way they had been raised. In this sense there can be continuity or conscious discontinuity with the family practices they have observed and experienced. Middleton (2011) suggests that being a mother enables young women 'to morally enact a caring role that was either similar to, or in opposition to, the care they had received from their own mothers' (2011, p. 234), and that this could be a process of reconnecting for some. Young women like Debbie, who are close to their mothers, talk about looking forward to having a baby because it means always having someone there, in the way that they have had their mother to talk to:

Just excitement, like when you're down or something, you know you've got someone there, haven't you, you know you've always got someone to talk to and, I don't know, you've always been close to your mam so you will be close to them.

Others, such as Haley, looked to their mothers as models to prove that it was possible to be a successful young mother and do well:

My mum is a young mum and she's done fine.

Some, such as Katy, had been estranged from her mother, and she was clear that she was going to raise her son in a different way to how she had been brought up. Earlier, she described how her childhood had been characterised by disruption, and she was determined to avoid this situation for her son. At the time of the first interview, she said that she did not want to have a relationship with anyone until Josh was older:

I don't think badly of my mum, but I wouldn't want Josh to think the way I do of my mum about me … there's been certain points of my life where I've hated my mum for putting men first and things like that, and I would never want Josh to think that I would do that, because I wouldn't. Because I've been there.

Having 'been there' for Katy meant having moved house and changed schools several times during her childhood, and she was also clear that she would not do that, mainly because it would mean taking Josh away from all the people he knew, as well as moving away from her support networks.

Mending Relationships

As Middleton (2011) observed, becoming a mother could lead to reconnection with their parents, particularly their mother, for some young people. At the first interview, Katy described her mother as 'not a hands on nana' and said that she did not see her much; however, 'not much' in this context was 'about once a week'. By the time of Katy's second inter-view six months later, things had changed, and whereas Katy's mother had previously wanted Josh to call her by her first name:

> She is nana now, she's very much nana now. Like, my mum will look after him and things for me, like if he's poorly and I don't want to take him into nursery, she'll look after him and things like that for me now, I don't even really have to ask.

Katy's pregnancy had also caused a rift between her and her father, and she described them as having nothing to say to each other because she felt that she had disappointed him. Yet once her son was born, the rift was healed very visibly within a week of the birth:

> I walked in and my dad went 'let's have a look then' and I was like 'there you go' (laughs) and I walked in the living room and he'd bought this Moses basket, he'd put this Moses basket out, he'd put the fire on, my dad never puts the fire on in the front room (laughs) and my dad had put this big coal fire on for him, and he'd like put some warm water in a jug ready to warm Josh's bottle up, and he had like nappies on the floor and a changing mat and everything, and he'd bought him some new like little tiny 'jamas and he'd put all that out for me and I kind of walked in and I was like 'hiya' and I was like 'I don't know what to do'. I felt really awkward and then he came in with like these presents for me and presents for Josh and I was like 'I don't know what to say' and he was just like 'is it alright if I have Josh for a bit?' and my dad just gave me a cuddle and from then on we've gone to my dad's pretty much every single Sunday and that's how it started.

Although this quote is quite long, I have included the full excerpt as it captures the hesitancy and awkwardness that Katy felt, and the effort that her father was making to welcome his new grandson into the family. Not only had he been shopping, he had lit a fire in the front room. In many homes, the front room is reserved for visitors and special occasions, so the significance of Katy's father lighting a coal fire in the front room should not be underestimated. Physically, by asking to hold the baby, and practi-cally, by buying things Katy will need, he bridges the difficulties they had experienced while she was pregnant, and mends their fragile relationship.

Becoming a Grandparent

As has been discussed previously, the announcement of a pregnancy by a teenager had most often been met by shock, disappointment and upset on the part of family members. However, the pregnancy and the baby were almost always regarded differently, with a baby being welcomed when the pregnancy had not been. Evidence shows parents and grandparents love and welcome the babies of teenage mothers (for example, Coleman and Cater 2006), and as Kirkman et al. (2001) found, 'a recurring theme in the interviews was of families unhappy with a teenage pregnancy becoming warm and loving when the grandchild was born' (2001, p. 288).

Some of the parents had been looking forward to becoming a grandparent as a natural and expected progression of family life. Sheila had been imagining becoming a grandmother even before her grandchild-to-be had been conceived, and this was a role to be thought of with pleasure:

> When we go for a walk around the park, and you see people with little ones, and we've always said 'wouldn't it be nice to have our own little grandchildren?'

Where Sheila had been anticipating her future grandchild, Debbie's grandmother Eileen and great-aunt Mary had not imagined Debbie being the first to have a baby. Nevertheless, they both spoke of the anticipated arrival with pleasure at various points in the interview:

Sheila	I have always wanted a grandchild for a long time, but I didn't think it would be Debbie, but then I did have a funny feeling she would be our first one to have one actually.
Debbie	Thanks!
Eileen	I never!
Sheila	Well no, because the boys haven't got girlfriends anyway so I knew, there's no signs off them, you know, but I did have a funny feeling she would be having one not long.
Mary	When she told me I said 'she's not!' because I never expected it.

Both Sheila and Debbie's father, Phil, talked about the grandchild bringing new life to the family, something that was important to them now their own children were grown up. Phil talked about the baby as someone to spoil and have fun with, and Debbie teased him as wanting a friend to watch TV with on a Friday night:

Phil   They've all grown up so obviously then they all get to the age where you don't see them anymore, now that there's going to be another little baby born, it will be like the same all over again, having your own kids again but the difference is we can give them back.

Mary   And you'll spoil that one more.

Phil   Well yeah. I'm looking forward to it, do you know what I mean.

For Sheila, part of the pleasure was because Debbie would continue to live with them once the baby was born, meaning that new life would come not only to the family, but to the home:

> So she's going to be living here and it will be quite exciting because they've all grown up now so it's like bringing life again, you know. (giggling)

In some cases, a younger child having a baby can present opportunities for being a grandparent that had previously been missed. Janet's older son had two children, but because his relationships with each of their mothers had ended, and there had been difficulties in access to his children for him and consequently for Janet, she had not seen her oldest grandchildren as they were growing up:

> I was looking forward, I've got two older grandchildren who because of the situation, I haven't, I didn't see them a lot when they were babies, and so I was looking forward to, sort of, like being there from day one and doing all the things that grandma gets to do all the time.

Although she had expressed her disappointment with her daughter for getting pregnant, she was clear throughout both interviews that she welcomed her new granddaughter, enjoyed being a grandmother, and was glad that Zara and the baby lived with her.

Perrier (2013) discusses 'generational right time' for becoming a grandparent, with her older respondents who had become mothers in their thirties, worrying that their children would not be able to have a relationship with grandparents because they were too old. They also saw it as a disadvantage that their parents might not be able to help with childcare, something Perrier points out is significant in the UK because a great deal of childcare for working parents is provided by grandparents. The younger mothers she interviewed emphasised both grandparental involvement in the child's life and the possibility of support for themselves as advantages to becoming a mother at a young age. Perrier spoke to parents but not grandparents; as Billings and Macvarish (2007) point out, the views and experiences of grandparents who are the parents of teen parents are under-researched, but what is known suggests that on the whole, intergenerational relationships are supportive, with some instances of tensions around the care that grandmothers give to their grandchildren. Like Sheila, Paula was looking forward to the arrival of her daughter Sarah's baby after having been very upset at first finding out about the pregnancy, as we heard earlier in Chapter 4. Paula already has twin grandchildren aged two, her older son and his girlfriend's children. Paula explained that as she had looked after her nephews and nieces, Sarah had always had babies around and therefore had some experience of childcare, but she would help without taking over:

> I'm always here, aren't I? On hand to help and advise, not that I'm gonna take over or anything, I just want Sarah to feel that she can come to me if she needs me … I've told her she can stay at home as much as she wants, but obviously she wants to be a family with her partner which is understandable, but she can stay at home as long as she wants.

Whereas Janet said she would be 'gutted' if Zara moved out with Ellie, Paula acknowledges that it is natural for Sarah to want her own home in due course, but here by repeating 'she can stay at home as long as she wants', seems to be suggesting that she would prefer it if she did not move out yet. She is also aware of the delicate balance between helping and taking over, possibly because her mother had taken over the care of her older sister's baby, born when Paula's sister was 15, so that she could finish her education. Paula had then started to look after her niece, had her own children, and then looked after her younger sister's child, born when her sister was 17, and supported her older niece who had twins when she was 19:

> As mine got older I started to take over the role of looking after the children, my sisters' children, while they worked, because they worked full-time so I tended to let them go and work which I did for my eldest sister, the one who had her daughter young. I looked after her and then she had another one five years ago and I looked after him, then she got him in nursery and then I looked after my other sister's youngest.

Being central to her family in terms of caring for children had meant that her sisters both had careers, but she now found herself unable to get a job at the age of 35; although she had passed exams at age 16, she had no work experience other than childcare within the family.

An aspect of generational right time, which in Perrier's study focusses on the age at which a woman becomes a mother, is the age at which a woman becomes a grandmother. This study reflects findings in Burton's (1990) study of a small community of African American mothers and grandmothers, and the concepts of accelerated family timetables and an age-condensed family structure, in that the four grandmothers interviewed became or were to become grandmothers between the ages of 32 and 41, and the two older women (Eileen and Mary) had become grandmothers in their thirties, with Paula's mother Cathy becoming a grandmother at 33. Both Eileen and Cathy had become great-grandmothers in their fifties. However, whilst Paula and Tina (grandmothers at 33 and 32) classed themselves as young grandmothers, Sheila, who would be 41 when Debbie's baby was born, did not:

SB   Do you think it makes a difference being a young grandma?
Eileen   No, she's older than I was (laughs).
Sheila   I'm 41 … that's an old age really for a grandma.
Eileen   I was 38, I think it was, with Kenny, wasn't I?
Mary   I think I was 34 when Laura was born, wasn't I?
Eileen   Yeah, you're 70-what now?
Mary   I'm 72.
Sheila   If I had my own way I'd have a baby myself but….

Sheila touches on an issue which for some of the other women in the study was a real one, that is, that they were still of childbearing age whilst their daughters were having children. Katy, for example, whose mother is 38, has four-year-old twin siblings. While Sheila laughed and shrugged at the unlikelihood of having another baby, and Eileen exclaimed 'ooh, no, I wouldn't!', those such as Katy's mother, in a new relationship, were having second or third children at the age at which the older mothers in Perrier's study, and typical middle-class women/career women, have their first.

The accelerated family timetables of Burton's (1990) study occurred because the people in her study perceived themselves to have a shorter than average life expectancy, therefore like the women in Geronimus' (2003) study could see no reason to postpone childbearing; indeed they may have felt an imperative to start a family early. Accelerated timetables also occurred due to an early end to adolescence for young people in that community, partly accounted for by taking on increased responsibility for the household and for childcare from around 14 years old. Many of the young women in this study had looked after small children: Katy and her twin siblings, Debbie and her cousin's twins, Haley and her older sister's babies. Others had grown up with their mothers looking after small children, so had been around small children and helped to care for them: Zara's mother Janet looking after the oldest of her grandchildren, Sarah's mother Paula caring for many of the younger children across the wider family. Only Naomi lacked experience in childcare before she had her son, with him being the first grandchild on both sides of the family. Where Burton's African American adolescents took on increased household responsibilities from around the age of 14, British working-class adolescents of earlier generations would have begun to earn a wage and contribute financially to the household after leaving school at 15 or 16.[1] Although most of the participants in this study were born after 1957 and therefore would have stayed at school until the age of 16 or older, many would have known people who were in work from the age of 15, and few of the older generation had remained at school beyond 16. Therefore,

---

[1] The 'school leaving age' in England and Wales was 15 until 1972, when it became 16; it changed to 17 in 2013. Although it is commonly referred to as school leaving age, in law it is the age at which a person can leave compulsory education; that education may not always take place in a school, with many 16- and 17-year-olds attending a college of further education.

accelerated timetables can be seen operating in the same way for British working-class adolescents as for African American adolescents, so that by the time they were in their late teens, they had accumulated several years' experience of responsible adulthood. In this cultural and social setting, having a child in late teens or very early twenties was not unusual, and did not seem young. Penny, one of advisors in Milton working with young people, who was in her late fifties, described how she left school at the age of 15 and went straight out to work:

> I was 15 when I left school, and a young 15, my birthday was June and then July I was working, and I got married at 20, which sounds really young but it didn't seem because like you say you'd have five years, and then had a child at 22, so I'd had seven years in work. … It wasn't a problem to me and it wasn't a problem to my family. In fact I was probably one of the maturer ones, they were usually having babies around the 19 mark.

Similarly, Joan in Seaborough had been working for two years by the time she got married at 18, and had her first child when she was 19. Their experiences illustrate what would now, in 2015, seem like accelerated transitions to adulthood but for their generation was not at all unusual.

As we have seen, in the UK and in other anglophone countries such as Canada and New Zealand, the average age of mothers is now 30. As far as participants in this study were concerned, several thought that a 'nice age' to have a baby is quite different, with Haley and Megan in Chapter 5 both saying that the early twenties was about right. Mary, aged 72, would seem to agree, as she is delighted that her 20-year-old granddaughter is going to make her a great-grandmother:

> My granddaughter, she's having one, there's only eight weeks between her and Debbie. She's 20 and when she rang me I said 'Oooh!' I said 'I'm over the moon!' (laughing).

Mary's comment about her granddaughter encapsulates a culture where it is normal and joyful to start a family by the age of 20. The difference between the teenagers having babies at the present time, and the older ones who had their children at roughly similar ages, such as Maureen, is that the current teenagers have not had the chance to bank several years' worth of work experience and earning power, partly due to changes in school leaving ages and patterns of employment, but also due to the fall in the number of jobs available to young people leaving education before the age of 18, or indeed 21.

Being a Family

As established earlier, 'being' a family is as much about family practices, 'doing' family, if not more so, than it is about particular structures or relationships. For the young women in the four families focussed on here, their family of origin was where they made their home, at least initially. Although Sarah said she planned to make a home with her partner and baby, she along with Haley, Debbie and Zara formed three-generation households with their parents and their child at the time of the study, or in Sarah and Debbie's cases, would form a three-generation household once the baby was born. In this sense they are not conforming to the norm discussed earlier of living in a household/nuclear family overlap. However, the teenagers and their babies are very much part of a family, as Phil, for example, said earlier when talking about 'bringing new life into the family'. Several of the families had conventional family structures, in terms of marriages/partnerships and living arrangements, in addition to talking about their families in much broader terms than the household/nuclear overlap. When Paula talked about her mother's relationships with grandchildren and great-grandchildren, she described a large extended family:

> She plays a great part in all the grandchildren and like the great-grandchildren because she has got others, because like my sister she was only 15 when she had her first, and their daughter has got twins as well. So (laughs) we have got a big expanded family, extended family but yeah she plays a great part in all the children's life, she's always been there for all of us, yeah always.

Although Paula and her sisters had moved houses, they had not moved far; the three sisters and their mother were all within walking distance or a short bus journey, so saw each other regularly. For both Paula and her mother, family practices had meant providing childcare not only for their own children, but also helping to raise their grandchildren and nieces and nephews. In terms of intergenerational transfers (Brannen 2003, 2006), at this point most of the transferring of resources is going to the younger generations, and mainly involves childcare; as Brannen points out, transfers tend to occur on gendered lines. For Paula, it has also meant sacrificing employability while her sisters developed their careers.

Naomi and Jamie were the most conventional of the young parents in terms of household/nuclear family overlap, with the financial support they received from their parents, who were guarantors for them which enabled them to rent their house, enabling this. They also received help with looking after their son once Naomi started her college course, with each grandmother looking after the baby for one day a week. As a result, they did not need to use any formal childcare. This meant that Naomi could go to the college she preferred, as the one that had a nursery did not offer a course she wanted to do, and the one where she wanted to study did not have a nursery. She was also happy that her baby was being cared for entirely within the family.

Debbie's baby would go to nursery for part of the week, but even before he is born, the family have worked out a schedule to look after him:

Sheila   The baby's going to go to the same college nursery because it's like I can't look after it, because like I work at school as well, you know, dinner ladying, so the times when Debbie is at college, he'll have to go into a nursery for a couple of days. I mean there's like, Thursday is your late day, isn't it?

Debbie   Yeah.

Sheila   Where she doesn't start until two so I could maybe work that round, I could maybe, then I'll leave work, I go out to work at like half past three so we still need someone to look after him....

Eileen   You know and I don't go to work until five.

Sheila   Yeah, so my mam can look after him until five....

Eileen   So there's always somebody there, you know—

Sheila   —That's it—

Eileen   —as long as I'm alright like.

Sheila   My mam could look after him until five and then, well until quarter to five and then I'd have to bring him home but he's going to be messing about. Will someone look after him again while I go back out to work till half past six?

Mary   Well, I'm only round the corner.

Sheila   Well, yeah, Mary has offered to help as well.

Two things are worth noting about this extract; firstly, the complex arrangements involving three generations: the baby's mother, grandmother, great-grandmother and great-aunt will be helping to care for him. Secondly, despite my question being addressed to Debbie, she only says one word in reply, and most of the answering is done by her mother. This raises the question of the extent to which Debbie will be able to work out her own way of being a mother, and the thin line between parents supporting and taking over.

Emotionally close and geographically close families enable the middle generation, the young parents, to pursue education and work opportunities, demonstrating that far from being the socially excluded individuals that policymakers think they are, young parents are very much socially included. Kinship networks operate to bring the new baby into the extended family, and enable the young parents to continue their education and eventually, find employment. As Hosie points out, teenage pregnancy is 'predominantly viewed as a negative end point in the trajectory of a young woman's life' (2007, p. 334). However, far from being an end to life chances, for the young people in this study parenthood is a natural, normal and welcomed stage in the life course, and as far as education and work is concerned, no more than a pause.

Different Shapes of Families, Different Ways of Doing Family

While the family discussed above are fairly conventional in terms of their composition and construction, one challenge for young mothers is how to construct their family if they are living with their parents, or no longer in a relationship with their baby's father. Where the young mother's parents are welcoming, this may help the young father to have a relationship with his baby and to continue his relationship with his girlfriend, even though he is not living with her. Phil, for example, talked about Gavin, Debbie's boyfriend, having to 'show responsibility now', and Shelia said:

> I've said he can stop when the baby's born and he can, he's not living here but he can help her out, maybe twice a week he could stop but that's it really.

However, although parents such as Sheila and Phil may be supportive, it is a challenge for young men to maintain their relationship in these circumstances, and to become a father. Megan, in South Wales, moved out of the family home into her own home with her partner when their baby was a year old, even though she knew it would be difficult financially:

> It was a big step ... I'm the type of person I'd rather have my own space. And it was easier for me to do stuff as myself as a young mother, to help Elen, than having my parents trying to tell me what to do and, you know. But yeah, I found it all right.

She and Owen, her partner, had maintained their relationship during the first year when they were not living together, and had, at the time of the interview, had their own home for four years.

For young women whose relationships have ended, parenting can become more complex if the baby's father wants to continue being involved, although this was only the case for one young woman in this study, Katy. Of the others who were interviewed, Zara and Haley knew that they would be raising their baby without the father's support from before the baby's birth (see Chapter 4 for details of this aspect of their stories). Amy's boyfriend had said he wanted to be involved but had only seen the baby once, shortly after the birth, and seven months later had not been in touch.

Like Sarah and Debbie, Haley had a close and supportive family, and both Haley and her mother could see advantages to raising her baby without the father's involvement, as they 'don't have to argue about who's having him on a weekend'. (The father had denied paternity, and refused to acknowledge in any way that he had any connection with Haley or her baby). Although

Haley planned to move out when she could find a flat nearby, Tina was adamant that she 'didn't want her going anywhere yet'. Throughout the interviews with Tina, and later with Haley and Tina, Haley's father Kevin was in the next room working on an extension to the kitchen, and came in and out of the interviews, or shouted comments from the kitchen, as below, that demonstrate closeness, warmth, and family humour:

Tina	Everybody in the family has said if they could get another baby like him they'd have one, they'd have another one.
Kevin	He's not hers anyway, he's ours! (shouted from the kitchen)
SB	It sounds as though he likes being a granddad. Do you like being a granddad?
Kevin	No! (Kevin's brother, helping with the DIY, laughs)
Tina	He says that all the time! He's like, 'I hate kids' and all the kids always go to him. He should be Father Christmas somewhere, shouldn't he?
Haley	Don't listen to granddad, he's a grumpy bum, isn't he?

What is noticeable about this exchange is not only the humour, but also the remark by Kevin that 'he's not hers, he's ours', in the light of what Haley had already said about his difficulty in accepting her pregnancy after the early deaths of other babies in the family.

Similarly Zara set out upon parenthood knowing she would be doing it without a partner, although with the support of her mother. Talking about the wider family, she said:

> Ellie doesn't have that much family, does she really? She has us, my aunty, my uncle, my granddad, my brother and my niece. That's it for her family.

Compared to the Baker, Jones and Smith families, this is a relatively small family, not least because of the estrangement between Zara and her father due to domestic violence, which had caused the break up in the relationship between Janet and Zara's father. So in that sense, Ellie is missing one-half of her potential relatives. Nevertheless, the family she does have is close knit, and by Zara's account, fond of her and generous with gifts.

Katy, who as we have seen has been brought closer to her parents since her son's birth, had a turbulent relationship with Josh's father Pete, marked by a number of separations and reunions. By the time she became involved in the study, she was clear that her relationship with Pete was over, not least because he had a son with a subsequent partner, and was now with a new girlfriend. Despite this, Katy talked very positively about him as a father, if not a partner:

> He's a brilliant dad, worst boyfriend in the world but he's a brilliant dad, he really is a brilliant dad, he's tried really hard for Josh and things like that, so in that respect I'm really proud of him because, well, Josh loves him. It's just, me and him are just a mess, that's all.

As far as Katy was concerned, although their arrangement might be unconventional, she was determined to make it work, for Josh's sake. As we saw earlier, she was very clear about not wanting Josh to have a similar childhood to herself, and determined to provide consistency for him. As such, she and Pete formed a family:

> We are a team, we are a family, we're not together but we are a family regardless and nobody can touch us as a family because me and Pete care about each other, we love each other, but I'm not in love with him and I don't want a relationship but we are a family.

At the second interview six months later, this was still working:

> This is what me and Pete both said we wanted when he was born really, we wanted him to know that we can be civil and we can be in the same room and stuff like that for him, like we do his parents evenings at nursery, we both go. Important things with doctors, we both go.

Thus, despite not following a conventional household/nuclear family pattern, Katy maintains family practices by describing what she and Pete do in terms of 'we are a family'. As argued by Morgan (1996) and Finch (2007), family here is a quality, and not a thing.

All the families in this chapter were close geographically, and in that way were similar to the families in the two East End studies (Young and Willmott 1962; Cornwell 1984), particularly in the sense of understanding distance. Young and Wilmott discuss a man who wanted the council to move him as far away as possible from his ex-wife, saying he would 'even go as far away as' somewhere which was about a five minute walk. When Sarah talked about getting her own home, she said she wanted to go back to where she came from, which was about a mile and a half away from where she lived; when Haley was asked if her sisters lived nearby she said no:

> One of my sisters lives on [two miles away] Road and my other sister lives on [three miles away] Lane, and both of them regret it so they want to move back up here.

Although two and three miles are not an easy walking distance in terms of popping in and out of each other's houses the way the East End families did, it is still a relatively short distance, and could be managed by bus. The Jones family were very like the families of the two East End studies as they described where each of them lived, roughly a five- to ten-minute walk from each other's houses. Geographical proximity is clearly important for maintaining intergenerational interaction (Hjalm 2012), but the way some of the participants talked about and perceived closeness in this study bears examination. Haley felt that two miles was not nearby, and for Sarah, going back to where she came from meant moving a mile and a half, while Katy refers to seeing her mother 'not much', which is once a week. Both geographical distance and temporal distance are compacted, so that people see each other frequently (at least once a week) and are within walking distance of much of their family (or if not, they want to be). Swedish research (Fors and Lennartsson 2008) suggests that this is class-related, with families where two generations are manual workers being much more likely to socialise frequently than families of non-manual workers. Although it is obvious that geographical closeness will determine frequency of meeting, it is the perceptions of closeness and distance that are interesting in the way Haley, Sarah and Katy speak.

Similarities and Differences Between the Generations

All the participants in this chapter were invited to take part because they had a similar characteristic, whichever generation they came from, that is, they had all been teenage mothers (and in some cases, teenage fathers). Apart from that, there were few similarities that could be applied broadly. In each generation, there were those who had had supportive parents despite their pregnancy (Mary, Sheila, Debbie; Sarah and Zara, Naomi and Jamie), and those who had not (Janet, Paula, Katy). Some had experienced stable childhoods while others had experienced disruption, violence or frequent house moves.

The main difference related to marriage, although not all the older participants had married: Sheila (aged 41) had; Paula (aged 35) had not. The generation above them had been married; Paula's mother Cathy was married at 18, and Sheila's aunt, Mary, had married at 17, and as she explained:

> I was married when he was born, because them days, it was a privilege of a man to marry you, well, morally.

Whereas Mary was already pregnant at the time of her wedding, Cathy was married before she conceived. Paula suggests that this made a difference in terms of how she was perceived, in terms of being a young mother:

> I think my mum was 18 going on 19 but she was married. It was different then, she was married, so I don't think it got frowned upon as much.

This encapsulates the shift in regarding teenage pregnancy as a moral problem due to the unmarried status of the mother to regarding it as a social problem because of the age of the mother. Because Cathy was married, being a mother at 18 was not a problem for that generation. Mary, being unmarried when she conceived, quickly married before her new husband went into the army and their son was born, thus solving the problem of potential immorality to become a married woman by the time her baby arrived.

The other question about what has changed over time relates to per-ceptions of what has changed rather than actual differences. As we saw earlier, in Chapter 2, the British public thinks that rates of teenage preg-nancy are much higher than they are (Ipsos MORI 2013), and the press talk about epidemics and high rates in a way that Lawlor and Shaw (2004) describe as a manufactured moral panic. Several of the interviewees said that not only was teenage pregnancy less frowned upon now, but that it was more common now than it had been, which is why it is less frowned upon, or, as Paula says, 'nobody batters an eyelid':

> There's more young mothers than there was when I was pregnant, there wasn't that many. It was more of a shock if you said you were pregnant, there was, like now if you go to schools there is a lot of young mums, isn't there? Whereas I recall when my sister was pregnant at 15 she was the only one in school pregnant, whereas now if you go to the school … There was far less teen pregnancies when I was younger. Whereas now I think it's just nobody batters an eyelid, do they?

Paula had her first child in 1998, which as has already been noted, was when the teenage pregnancy rate had been falling steadily for 30 years, even though the issue was about to be highlighted by the TPS. As has also been noted, the rate has been falling steadily ever since, so there are in fact far fewer teenage pregnancies at the time of this interview than when Paula had her first baby, not more. Sheila also said that there are more pregnant teenagers now than when she had her oldest son 26 years ago. This raises the question of why people's perceptions are so far from reality. From Lawlor and Shaw's perspective, this is due to the media manufac-turing the stories, either in order to encourage a moral panic, or as Tyler argues, as part of a process of labelling one group in society as 'national abjects' (2013, p. 9) who then become scapegoats for society's ills.

Views about changes in behaviour may also have more to do with per-ceptions of how people used to behave, than actual changes:

Eileen Like you had to, you didn't have to get married but it was a thing where you knew you had to, you couldn't have a baby out of wedlock, put it that way.

Mary   And they didn't believe in living together like they do in today's world.

Eileen   You daren't sleep together, that wasn't allowed, but it has changed completely.

Here, Mary mentions the major social change in the period between her youth and Debbie's, which is that couples are now more likely to live together than get married. The most recent data for the UK shows that cohabiting couples are the fastest growing family type (ONS 2015), and this change is not confined to the UK; marriage rates have been decreasing in the USA for decades, and the number of births taking place to unmarried mothers compared to married mothers has been increasing in the US and across Europe (Luker 1996; Furstenberg 2007), not just in the UK.

What is also notable about this quote is that Eileen says sleeping together was not allowed, while sitting next to her sister who had slept with her boyfriend before marriage, in 1955. People's perceptions about what is or was true, and what actually happened, are clearly very different even when the evidence that they are not is sitting next to them at the dining table.

Conclusions

This chapter has examined the way families react to the arrival of a new baby when the parent is a teenager, and the grandparents are relatively young having been teenage parents themselves. The concept of family has been used in a broad way to include not just members of a nuclear family or a household, but to encompass grandparents, great-grandparents, siblings, aunts and other relatives. Mitchell and Green (2002) suggest that although the idea of an extended and supportive family is often portrayed as a historically cosy image, rather than an everyday reality of the twenty-first century, close kinship networks are still pivotal in the lives of many young mothers. Although it is not always a simple relationship, particularly as families take on different formations, the evidence in this chapter makes it clear that supportive family networks are important for many young parents. Whether or not the timing was ideal, there was an expectation that young women would become mothers, and the older generation would become grandparents at some point in their lives. This was seen as a natural and normal progression, and something to be anticipated, usually with pleasure. As McDermott and Graham (2005) found, families provided practical and financial support for the young parents, including housing and childcare. In addition, the older generation provided emotional support, particularly by validating them as doing something worthwhile for the family by providing the next generation, which may have acted as a buffer against the stigmatising and judgemental encounters occurring outside the home.

The young people in the study had a mix of backgrounds in terms of family life; although most had experienced a stable upbringing with both birth parents, some had experienced violence in the family, divorce of parents, or mothers with unstable relationship histories or a history of drug abuse. As in Middleton's research (Middleton 2011), young parents' histories could influence their parenting experience: a few were very keen to be a different type of mother to their own mother, whilst many looked to their mothers and sisters as examples of how to succeed. As in Mitchell and Green's study (2002), several of the young mothers relied on their mothers for support. Whereas most of the young people had strong aspirations to what might be described as traditional family life—settling down with a partner in their own home—others, who were no longer in intimate relationships with their baby's father, were content, for now at least, to be a single parent. This incorporated those who, though living apart, continued to parent together. Several young mothers continued to live with their mother or both parents, in a multigenerational household. Within the context of the wider family, grandparents-to-be were enthusiastic about a new baby, even if they had not been enthusiastic about the pregnancy. In this sense, the young mother takes up a valued role within the family, being one who is bringing new life, and the next generation, to the family. Almost all the young people reported that they had supportive families, and in one case where there had been estrangement prior to the arrival of the baby, having a new grandson had brought one father close to his teenage daughter again.

Given the mix of structures and the ways in which participants talked about family, both in terms of who comprised family, and what various members did, it is clear that families are, as Morgan says, best described as sets of activities and not structures. It is also apparent that for many working-class families, the geographical and temporal relationships have not changed a great deal in terms of activities since the 1950s and 1960s. Rates of teenage parenting and marriage are lower in the 2010s than 60 years ago, but family practices are much the same in the way that families, especially the women in those families, carry out day-to-day care, offer support, and form kinship networks that are socially inclusive. As Jamieson (1999) points out, we need to understand the practical and material circumstances of people's lives in order to place relationships into their social and economic contexts. Many of the young people could work or study only because they had the support of other relatives who themselves might be working, with more than one job in some cases. None of the young parents could be described as well off financially, but the strong, caring kinship networks that existed for them meant that despite living in areas characterised as socially excluded, they themselves were part of something that had meaning and significance for all participants.

References

Billings, J. R., & Macvarish, J. (2007). *Teenage parents' experiences of parenthood and views of family support services in Kent. Service Users Report, Postnatal.* Canterbury: Centre for Health Services Studies, University of Kent.

Boden, J. M., Fergusson, D. M., & Horwood, L. J. (2008). Early motherhood and subsequent life outcomes. *Journal of Child Psychology and Psychiatry, 49,* 151–160.

Brannen, J. (2003). Towards a typology of intergenerational relations: Continuities and change in families. *Sociological Research Online, 8*(2). Retrieved September 30, 2015, from http://www.socresonline.org.uk/8/2/brannen.html

Brannen, J. (2006). Cultures of intergenerational transmission in four-generation families. *The Sociological Review, 54*(1), 133–154.

Burton, L. (1990). Teenage childbearing as an alternative life-course strategy in multigeneration black families. *Human Nature, 1*(2), 123–143.

Chase-Lansdale, P. L., Brooks-Gunn, J., & Zamsky, E. S. (1994). Young African-American multigenerational families in poverty: Quality of mothering and grandmothering. *Child Development, 65*(2), 373–393.

Coleman, L., & Cater, S. (2006). 'Planned' teenage pregnancy: Perspectives of young women from disadvantaged backgrounds in England. *Journal of Youth Studies, 9*(5), 595–616.

Cornwell, J. (1984). *Hard earned lives; accounts of health and illness from East London.* London: Tavistock.

Deleire, T., & Kalil, A. (2002). Good things come in threes: Single-parent multigenerational family structure and adolescent adjustment. *Demography, 39*(2), 393–413.

Dunifon, R., & Kowaleski-Jones, L. (2007). The influence of grandparents in single-mother families. *Journal of Marriage and Family, 69*, 465–481.

Finch, J. (2007). Displaying families. *Sociology, 41*(1), 65–81.

Fors, S., & Lennartsson, C. (2008). Social mobility, geographical proximity and intergenerational family contact in Sweden. *Ageing and Society, 28*(2), 253–270.

Furstenberg, F. (2007). *Destinies of the disadvantaged. The politics of teenage childbearing.* New York: Russell Sage Foundation.

Geronimus, A. T. (2003). Damned if you do: Culture, identity, privilege, and teenage childbearing in the United States. *Social Science and Medicine, 57*, 881–893.

Geronimus, A. T., & Korenman, S. (1992). The socioeconomic consequences of teen childbearing reconsidered. *The Quarterly Journal of Economics, 107*(4), 1187–1214.

Geronimus, A. T., & Korenman, S. (1993). Maternal youth or family background? On the health disadvantages of infants with teenage mothers. *American Journal of Epidemiology, 137*, 213–225.

Gibb, S. J., Fergusson, D. M., Horwood, J., & Boden, J. M. (2014). Early motherhood and long-term economic outcomes: Findings from a 30-year longitudinal study. *Journal of Research on Adolescence, 25*(1), 163–172.

Goodman, C. C. (2007). Family dynamics in three-generation grandfamilies. *Journal of Family Issues, 28*(3), 355–379.

Hjalm, A. (2012). 'Because we know our limits': Elderly parents' views on intergenerational proximity and intimacy. *Journal of Aging Studies, 26*, 296–308.

Hosie, A. C. S. (2007). 'I hated everything about school': An examination of the relationship between dislike of school, teenage pregnancy and educational disengagement. *Social Policy and Society, 6*(3), 333–347.

Hotz, V. J., McElroy, S. W., & Sanders, S. G. (1996). The costs and consequences of teenage childbearing for mothers. *Chicago Policy Review, 64*, 55–94.

Hunter, A. (1997). Counting on grandmothers: Black mothers' and fathers' reliance on grandmothers for parenting support. *Journal of Family Issues, 18,* 251–269.

Ipsos MORI. (2013). *Perils of perception.* London: Survey for Royal Statistical Society and King's College.

Jamieson, L. (1999). Intimacy transformed? A critical look at the 'pure relationship'. *Sociology, 33*(3), 477–494.

Kirkman, M., Harrison, M., Hillier, L., & Pyett, P. (2001). 'I know I'm doing a good job': Canonical and autobiographical narratives of teenage mothers. *Culture, Health and Sexuality, 3*(3), 279–294.

Lawlor, D., Mortensen, L., & Nybo Andersen, A. M. (2011). Mechanisms underlying the associations of maternal age with adverse perinatal outcomes: A sibling study of 264,695 Danish women and the firstborn offspring. *International Journal of Epidemiology, 40,* 1205–1214.

Lawlor, D. A., & Shaw, M. (2004). Teenage pregnancy rates: High compared with where and when? *Journal of the Royal Society of Medicine, 97*(3), 121–123.

Lee, E., Clements, S., Ingham, R., & Stone, N. (2004). *A matter of choice? Explaining national variation in teenage abortion and motherhood.* York: Joseph Rowntree Foundation.

Luker, K. (1996). *Dubious conceptions: The politics of teenage pregnancy.* Cambridge: Harvard University Press.

Macvarish, J. (2010). The effect of 'risk-thinking' on the contemporary construction of teenage motherhood. *Health, Risk & Society, 12*(4), 313–322.

McDermott, E., & Graham, H. (2005). Resilient young mothering: Social inequalities, late modernity and the 'problem' of 'teenage' motherhood. *Journal of Youth Studies, 8*(1), 59–79.

Middleton, S. (2011). 'I wouldn't change having the children - not at all'. Young women's narratives of maternal timing: What the UK's Teenage Pregnancy Strategy hasn't heard. *Sexuality Research and Social Policy, 8,* 227–238.

Mitchell, W., & Green, E. (2002). 'I don't know what I'd do without our Mam' motherhood, identity and support networks. *The Sociological Review, 50,* 1–22.

Morgan, D. H. J. (1996). *Family connections: An introduction to family studies.* Cambridge: Polity.

Morgan, D. H. J. (2013). *Rethinking family practices.* Basingstoke: Palgrave Macmillan.

Office for National Statistics. (2015). *Statistical bulletin: Families and households 2014.* London: Stationery Office.

Perrier, M. (2013). No right time: The significance of reproductive timing for younger and older mothers' moralities. *The Sociological Review, 61*(1), 69–87.

Smith, D. E. (1993). The standard North American family: SNAF as an ideological code. *Journal of Family Issues, 14*(3), 50–65.

SmithBattle, L. (1996). Intergenerational ethics of caring for teenage mothers and their children. *Family Relations, 45*, 56–64.

SmithBattle, L. (1997). Continuity and change in family caregiving practices with young mothers and their children. *Image – Journal of Nursing Scholarship, 29*, 145–149.

SmithBattle, L. (2000). Developing a caregiving tradition in opposition to one's past: Lessons from a longitudinal study of teenage mothers. *Public Health Nursing, 17*, 85–93.

SmithBattle, L. (2006). Family legacies in shaping teen mothers' caregiving practices over 12 years. *Qualitative Health Research, 16*, 1129–1144.

Thomson, R. (2000). Dream on: The logic of sexual practice. *Journal of Youth Studies, 3*(4), 407–427.

Tyler, I. (2013). *Revolting subjects: Social abjection and resistance in neoliberal Britain*. London: Zed Books.

Young, M., & Willmott, P. (1962). *Family and kinship in East London*. Harmondsworth: Penguin.

7

'There's a Pattern Going on There': Local Contexts of Teenage Parenting

This chapter discusses the findings from the focus groups and interviews with staff in the various locations of the study. People taking part included youth workers, key workers in teenage pregnancy and parenting support services including a young dads' worker, a family nurse practitioner, specialists in sexual health, community development workers, Connexions staff, team managers, a former Sure Start Plus manager, and people working on service commissioning in local authorities. Talking to this range of people, who have accumulated many years' experience in the field, provided perspectives on the cultural context of young parenting in their areas, as well as insights into how services can best be provided to support young parents, that to date have rarely been presented. The appendix provides further information about participants and their roles in each location; all names have been changed to maintain anonymity.

Although there is literature on the support services used and required by teenage parents, it tends to focus on the young people themselves (for example, Yardley 2009), and there is very little published literature on research with professionals who work with young parents. McLeod et al. (2006) looked at whether formal support networks promoted

© The Editor(s) (if applicable) and The Author(s) 2016

157

S. Brown, *Teenage Pregnancy, Parenting and Intergenerational Relations*,
DOI 10.1057/978-1-137-49539-6_7

social inclusion amongst teenage mothers, and although they found that service providers were keen to take a holistic approach in advising and supporting young mothers, it was unclear whether formal services promoted the development of social support networks amongst the young parents. Kidger (2004) also questioned whether policy approaches could develop social support and promote social inclusion using formal services as a vehicle. However, since McLeod et al.'s study was carried out, there have been two changes in government in the UK (from Labour to a Conservative and Liberal Democrat coalition in May 2010, followed by the General Election in May 2015 resulting in a Conservative government), and both governments made cuts to public spending which have led to reductions in service provision. These have included cuts to Sure Start and Sure Start Plus services and a narrowing of the role of the Connexions service, which has limited their ability to provide a holistic approach, as well as limiting the range of services and support they can provide. Malin and Morrow (2009) explored the role of Sure Start Plus advisors, and found that having a professional with a dedicated role of supporting young parents was valuable, both for young people and as a way of bringing institutional support together. However, the focus on individual empowerment within the TPS and the emphasis on economic participation as a measure of social inclusion, do not address the influence of social structures on the ability of individuals to make what are perceived from a policy point of view as rational choices. Austerberry and Wiggins (2007) argue that disregarding the wider socio-economic context within which young parents operate puts expectations on young mothers which are essentially setting them up to fail.

Parenting programmes, usually aimed at parents living in areas of high socio-economic deprivation or labelled as 'troubled', have become increasingly popular as a policy solution to the notion of problem families. For the Coalition government, the Troubled Families programme (DCLG 2012a, 2012b) became a key plank of family-related social policy, and it has been extended by the Conservative government. Although this is a problematic and much challenged notion, it has persisted, largely based on the argument that an underclass of people exist, and their existence persists not least because of cycles of poor parenting (Murray 1990). In the UK, it can be dated from initiatives introduced by Keith Joseph, cabinet member in the Thatcher governments from 1979–1986, having previously been Secretary of State for Social Services from 1970 to 1974. Shortly after the Conservative government's election defeat of 1974, Joseph made a speech (Joseph 1974) arguing that cycles of deprivation were due to mothers of low intelligence and low educational attainment having too many children. Despite the controversy stirred up by the speech, the concept of cycles of deprivation, and the idea that poverty is caused by inadequate mothers having too many children, have persisted in approaches to social policy in the UK, as we have seen in earlier chapters.

However, little evidence exists to show how and why parenting programmes work, if indeed they do; a systematic review conducted by Coren et al. (2003) found that the types of programmes studied in much of the research they reviewed were too diverse for them to make robust conclusions about the value of the programmes. Furthermore, many programmes, and all those included in Coren et al.'s review, focus solely on teenage mothers, despite evidence that it is beneficial to include young fathers (Moran et al. 2004; Ferguson and Gates 2015). A problem with Coren et al.'s review is that one inclusion factor for a study was that it was about a programme aimed at teenage mothers defined as all under 20; no distinction was made between younger and older teenagers, despite evidence that suggests the detrimental outcomes listed by Coren et al. as associated with teenage parenting are more likely to be associated with very young parents, that is, mothers aged 14 and below.

As described in Chapter 3, the primary location for the study, Seaborough, had featured regularly as one of the teenage pregnancy hotspots throughout the life of the TPS, although rates of pregnancy particularly for the very young teens had fallen dramatically. The other locations in England were local authorities which were statistical neighbours of Seaborough, two in the north-west and one on the south coast. In addition, a location in each of Scotland and Wales that have also experienced high rates of teen pregnancy were included. Many of the staff had worked in Teenage Pregnancy Support Units set up as part of the TPS, and although the strategy itself was no longer in place and service provision had been reorganised by the local authority, they continued to do the same sort of work albeit within a different organisational structure. Staff in these locations therefore have a great deal of experience over a number of years in working with young parents and parents-to-be, and provide insights into local cultures in terms of 'what it's like round here' for young people. Most of the staff interviewed were not providing parenting programmes of the sort discussed above, although one of the Scottish interviewees was a family nurse practitioner whose role was to provide intensive one-to-one support with a small case load of young parents. The role of most of the participants we hear from in this chapter was to provide ongoing support to young parents via drop-in sessions, support groups and occasional home visits, and through running advice sessions or providing one-to-one advice on issues such as housing, benefits, education and training, and employment.

In this chapter I present and discuss the findings from the interviews and focus groups with the staff members. Connections are made between what the staff said, and what the teenagers and their families said, in order to draw some conclusions about the influence of local cultures on teenage pregnancy and parenting.

Understanding Fertility and Contraception

As discussed in Chapter 4, young women can lack knowledge about fertility, pregnancy and contraception, and also may not be fully aware of the range of methods of contraception available, or how they work. It can also be a difficult process of trial and error for young women to find a method that suits them (Jewell et al. 2000). Several of the nurses and youth workers suggested that some young women had a poor understanding of reproductive biology and their own fertility, which may have contributed to unplanned pregnancies:

> I do the basics of little diagrams of a 28-day cycle, explaining to them how their cycle works, some of these girls don't even understand that. So even though they're studying biology some of them, they still don't understand how their cycle works. (Moira, Bridgetown)

Sandra   And some of them really don't understand about reproduction, they kind of think that you have your period and then you're alright to have sex for three weeks.

Joan   Yeah, they're very unaware of their own bodies, aren't they, a lot.
(Seaborough)

Lack of understanding about how contraception worked, combined with
poor advice about potential problems particularly with taking the pill,
was also felt to contribute:

> Most of mine are down to contraception mishaps, being on the pill and
> they've not received the proper advice in the first place, that if you're sick or
> if you are on antibiotics or if you miss a pill or if you are not regular, then
> you may get caught pregnant. And a lot of them are quite naive and the
> doctors, to be honest, do not give out, they hand the tablets over but they
> don't tell them face to face actually these are the risks. (Elaine, Seaborough)

Previous studies (Brown and Guthrie 2010; Falk et al. 2010; Pratt et al.
2014) have found that young women are often unaware that an upset
stomach (specifically, vomiting within two hours of taking the pill), irregular use and irregular periods can affect the effectiveness of the contraceptive pill. Despite guidance from the Faculty of Sexual Health (2012)
that the majority of antibiotics do not cause oral contraceptives to fail,
it is clear from Elaine's comment above that there is still some confusion about the relationship between antibiotics and the pill. Frost et al.'s
(2012) American study asked young people, men and women, about
contraceptive knowledge and found that over half the young men and
quarter of young women lacked knowledge about contraceptive methods, and that lack of knowledge was linked to risky behaviour. Sahili
et al.'s (2002) study in Scotland is interesting in that it asks young (aged
11–15) teenagers about intended contraceptive use, as part of a survey
about knowledge and sex education, but it then asks pregnant teenagers
(aged 14–16) about actual use. Whereas almost all the first group said
that they would use contraception, 71 per cent of the pregnant teenagers had not been using contraception regularly, and only 4 per cent were
using anything at the time of conception. The gap appears to be in practical knowledge: although the first group intended to use contraception,
73 per cent of girls and 52 per cent of boys were aware of available services leaving a sizeable number who were not. Most girls knew about
emergency contraception, but only 59 per cent of boys did, and a third

of the teens felt that they did not receive adequate sex education. The authors argue that young men's lack of knowledge in particular could have an impact on the ability of young people to have safe sex.

Sex education in the UK is compulsory in maintained schools, but it is part of the science curriculum, so lessons often focus solely on biological aspects of reproduction. Lessons may not address issues such as relationships and the complexities of managing and negotiating contraception. Research with young people has found that they dislike the emphasis on biology and would prefer a much broader curriculum covering sex and relationships in a more holistic, non-biological way (Forrest et al. 2004). It seems from some of the comments made both by staff and young people that the focus on science is not always that helpful to young people, indeed it appears that they may not necessarily understand how their bodies work despite having biology lessons. In addition, although provision of sex education is compulsory, attendance is not, and parents may opt to withdraw their child from the lesson. Furthermore, if there are only one or two lessons, or if, as in some schools, a speaker is brought in from an outside agency to do a one-off talk, any young person not at school on that day will miss out. This was felt to be a factor by some of the staff members:

> The ones that aren't accessing schools, it's your low attenders and things like that, the ones that skip school, they're the ones I feel are missing that education bit. (Elaine, Seaborough)
>   If you're a bit naughty or if you're excluded from the school you don't have them [PSHE lessons], which is ridiculous. (Bernie, Carville)

Poor sex education and lack of knowledge about reproduction and fertility were seen as key contributing factors to teenage conceptions, despite the emphasis on biology in the curriculum. It seems, then, that many teenagers are being given sex education that not only fails to meet their wishes in terms of issues around relationships and feelings, it also fails to meet their needs in terms of understanding their own bodies.

Education

Education as a whole was seen as an important factor, both in terms of school attendance prior to pregnancy, and the role of education for young women once they become pregnant and then a parent. Some connected lack of engagement with school and poor attendance with pregnancy rates, and some evidence indicates that young women who have unplanned pregnancies are more likely to be truanting or excluded from school prior to pregnancy (Scottish Parliament 2013):

Tracy   The link with truancy is massive.
SB   Truancy?
Tracy   Yeah massive, practically every single young parent I have worked with will say 'oh, I never really went mainstream', didn't really go like that, or 'I went but I had a laugh while I was in isolation most of the time'. (Barton)

> We've looked at all of our girls that were referred in 2012 … of the school age ones, 80 per cent of them had attendance problems, that's the biggest dominant risk factor, not being in school or not having education welfare involved, all that sort of thing. (Simon, Norland)

As well as lack of attendance at school being a factor leading up to the pregnancy, once a young woman was pregnant and had a baby, re-engagement with education was much less likely:

> What the girls were telling us was once they missed school, they got onto the treadmill of disengagement, and then when they were pregnant it was like the straw that broke the camel's back. In terms of engagement with education, a year out and then that was it really, they weren't ever back in as such. (Ian, Barton)

As highlighted by Vincent and Thomson (2010), the attitude of the school is very influential in terms of whether a young woman is allowed to carry on her education at her school if she becomes pregnant. A young women who has been a diligent pupil and who is seen as a good student is more likely to be able to remain at school; those who were disengaged by the time they got pregnant were more likely to be sent to a pupil referral unit or be home schooled, whether or not this was what they wanted:

Simon   So it's that strength of will, I suppose, of people who want to [stay at school]. And I mean it's about, the classic example is how a school treats a girl who gets pregnant at school age. If that young woman is an achiever they'll support her.

Carol   They'll keep them up.

Simon   They'll give her a load of homework, they'll help her out. If that young woman was off anyway before she was pregnant they want to get rid straightaway. And I think that's the problem.

Ingrid   Yeah, it is.

Some schools prefer pregnant teenagers to move out of mainstream education into a special unit, sometimes citing the health and safety of the young woman as the reason, and sometimes, it was suggested by some of Vincent and Thomson's respondents, because having a pregnant pupil at school might tarnish the reputation of the school.

In some areas, colleges could offer better opportunities to young parents to enable them to continue in education, both in terms of offering on-site child care, and also allowing flexibility in attendance, which could make allowances if, for example, a child was ill:

> Our college of further education has really done some fantastic work in terms of accommodating the needs of teenage parents more and more, so that in some respects they're kind of pushing the boat out a lot further than the schools. And they're just being really flexible about curriculum, so you can be out for a while and then back in and still do the courses, so it's providing opportunities. (Ian, Barton)

There seemed to be a great deal of variation in approaches to education across the localities, with some examples of very good practice which aimed to support young parents to continue their education. American and Canadian research (Kelly 2000; Luttrell 2003; Gregson 2009) shows that flexibility and supportive structures that take into account the challenges faced by young mothers are critical in enabling them to complete their schooling.

Reactions to Pregnancy

As discussed earlier, a very small minority of the teenagers interviewed had planned their pregnancy, most being unplanned, and the experience of people working with young parents bore this out:

> About 99.9 per cent unplanned. I've come across one or two in the five years that have actually planned it. (Karen, Milton)

The discussions with families showed that although the vast majority of teenage pregnancies were unplanned, a baby was not necessarily unwanted, and the experiences of many of the staff members concurred with this:

> I would say the majority of pregnancies are not planned. But that doesn't then mean that they're not wanted, you know, once they realise they're pregnant I would say that in the main they are happy to continue. (Clare, Bridgetown)

As we saw in Chapter 6, a common reaction to the announcement, or discovery, of the pregnancy by the teenagers' parents was shock and upset, and a feeling that they had wished for 'something better' for their daughters. However, a new baby was usually seen as a welcome addition to the family, something Clare, a Family Nurse Practitioner, had seen in the families she worked with:

> Very quickly they do come round, you know, the baby and the new generation, and it's very much accepted and loved once they get over that initial shock.

Families were often geographically close, so a young mother would probably have several female relatives within easy reach, who themselves had experienced parenthood at a young age, and who, on the whole, were supportive:

> Well, it's not a dreadful thing, it's a baby, isn't it? It's kind of hard, because it is a blessing to a lot of families, isn't it? It's exciting, it's really positive, so it's kind of balancing those emotions anyway. (Ingrid, Norland)

As Kirkman et al. (2001) found, a new baby is welcomed into the family by the grandparents, even though they may have expressed shock and disappointment about the pregnancy at first. In addition, in many cases (all the cases as far as the interviewees in this study were concerned) it was not the first time there had been a teenage pregnancy in the family:

> We're not talking about the first time this has happened in families, so yes there's a degree of normality. (Clare, Bridgetown)
>
> In some families it's kind of more acceptable for them to have a baby at a younger age. That's a controversial thing to say but for some of them it is okay and it's tradition within the family that maybe mum had a child at a younger age, and so they're supported. (Nancy, Milton)

Age at first birth is differentiated by class and education, a differentiation which is becoming wider (Smith and Ratcliffe 2009); people from working-class backgrounds have tended to start their families at a younger age than people from middle-class backgrounds, and this is closely linked with educational attainment and possibly with the difference in impact on future earnings of the timing of having children. Smith and Ratcliffe (2009) highlight the 'increasing divergence in family and working lives between women who have post-compulsory education and those who do not' (2009, p. 41), and suggest that there is greater polarisation in age of childbearing due to education. There is also, of course, polarisation in employment opportunities due to education, and where a young woman sees that employment opportunities are limited, motherhood may be appealing as a way of gaining a sense of achievement:

> I feel it comes back to what expectations people have of themselves and their lives, and how they're going to pan out. And also that I suppose pregnancy can sometimes be seen as a success in life, in maybe a life that's not going to have many other potential successes in it, and it's something that you've done and that you can do, and that you can show somebody else that you've achieved. And, you know, that kind of makes it difficult to change culture, because it feels like it's a cultural thing in this area. (Rose, Bridgetown)

Marion also felt that there was a culture in her area of 'the way it's always been done', in the sense that young women were more likely to model themselves on their own mothers than on a life they know little about:

> It's the way it's always been done and this is it, they're just repeating history. … But the difficulty is because there is nothing out there to aspire to, the jobs, okay, they could go to university, they could get a degree, there's no guarantee they'll get a job. So their aspiration, they aspire to be like their mothers rather than aspiring to be like somebody else that's done better, because that's more realistic. (Marion, Carville)

The group discussions considered the way in which young people's aspirations seemed limited not only by staying with what they knew, but also by what was expected of them by others, particularly their families:

Lesley   In the more affluent areas young people do tend to have higher aspirations, the parents tend to have higher aspirations for them, so they're encouraged to continue with that education and not to have children. Whereas in the more deprived areas it's, well, what are you going to do when you finish school at 16 or 18, because, 'well, I went working in Tesco's' or 'I went doing this and I had you when I was 18 so I couldn't go to university'. I think there is a very, there's still a very stark difference in socio-economic statuses.

Jill   Yeah, across the borough, yeah definitely.

Penny   I certainly just work in the same patch over and over; I never go out to the affluent areas. (Milton)

Staff in several of the locations felt that the aspirations a young person has are influenced by the area they come from, and there is a close connection to levels of deprivation. As Rose said above, the expectations they have for themselves of how they see their lives developing. In all the groups, it was possible to identify a difference between areas within the same city:

> There are issues which often seem linked to aspiration, where 'I am seeing myself as a mother' or 'I'm seeing myself as someone who's going to go to college', and you've got that kind of split happening. And it is marked

[across the two sides of the city] ... it's very strong, it's probably four or five times different. (Ian, Barton)

However, although the desire to be a parent at a young age may seem to be a sign of limited aspirations for those not achieving in school, becoming a young parent can lead to a desire to achieve more in life and return to education, not least because the young parent now has someone to care for, and someone for whom they have responsibility. In this sense, young parenthood can, for many young people, become a turning point in their lives.

Parenthood as a Turning Point

Earlier chapters discussed how some young people saw becoming a parent as a turning point, and many staff members across all the locations made the same argument. As we saw earlier, many young parents said that they had ambitions to do well now that they had a child to bring up, and many of them had returned to education or taken up education or training if they had previously fallen out of the system:

> Loads of the young parents that I work with have seen it as a turning point in their life, to take that responsibility, to turn their life around or to have a go at making something a little bit different. So sometimes obviously you've got the other side of the coin that Jon was talking about earlier, where people won't take responsibility, but for a lot of them it is a turning point. It's a way to become more included. (Tracy, Barton)

It is interesting to note that Tracy here says that parenthood is a way to become more included; as discussed earlier, the prevailing policy view is that teenage parenthood leads to social exclusion, whilst a substantial amount of qualitative research suggests the opposite (Graham and McDermott 2006). Interviews with the young people showed that many of them had become more involved with education, and with health and welfare support services, which suggests that they are becoming more engaged with the services that will enable them to avoid the NEET label.

Another way in which parenthood could be a turning point was in the way it enables young people to make a life for themselves and their child that is different from the way they have grown up:

> With some of mine it's made their lives better, they've got away from the dreadful family life they were brought up with and they are determined that their child is not going to have the life that they had, and it's actually improved their way of living, I've got a couple like that, it's actually saved them having a child, it's given them a better life. (Elaine, Seaborough)

Becoming a parent provides an opportunity, and an incentive, to change and to become a different person:

> When young parents are on the cusp of a change, quite a lot of the time they'll say 'right, I want to get out of here. Everyone knows my business, I'm fed up of it, I can't live in that area anymore, I just get dragged down by this, I get dragged down by that, I'm always getting involved in this and that.' (Tracy, Barton)

Whereas prior to becoming pregnant, education had often been a negative experience for many young parents, once they had a baby their views often changed. Having responsibility for a baby provided an incentive to re-engage with the education system:

> I think they probably had issues at school, but now they're more inclined to think all right, fresh start, I'll go to college. (Anne, Barton)

This is consistent with much of the research on this topic, which is predominantly North American. Kelly (2000), Luttrell (2003) and Gregson (2009) all found that the teachers and other staff who worked with the pregnant and parenting teens in their studies presented education as a responsibility, with 'messages of social redemption and educated motherhood' (Luttrell 2003, p. 23) focussing on how young women should complete their education for their baby's sake. However, this message was not pushed onto an unreceptive audience; as in those studies and in this one, young parents were keen to return to an interrupted education if their pregnancy had resulted in a break, or as Anne says above, make a fresh start if they had previously been disengaged.

Support for getting back into education includes Care to Learn, which provides childcare until a young person is 19. However, some young parents found that just as they were at a stage when they could contemplate going to college, they were no longer eligible for support, a finding echoed in Canadian research (Shoveller et al. 2011). The Milton focus group, which included Lesley and Zoe who worked for Connexions, discussed this problem at length, and participants felt that services should be extended to support people up to the age of 21, or even 25:

Lesley   Because we speak to a lot of 19-year-olds but then it's almost too late for them to get Care to Learn because they have to be 19 when they go on the course. A lot of 19-year-olds will come back to us, and they're wanting support and they're wanting that, then they're out of our range. And I think for some of those, they do need a bit more support from us and from different agencies.

Nancy   It's like, what do we do with ourselves now?

Yasmin   We're only supposed to have under twenties in our group but I have bent the rules a bit, we have got a 20 and a 21-year-old.

Penny   I was just going to say, we work from ten to 19 but if they're vulnerable we'd go up to 25.

Lesley   Well, we only go up to 25 with—

Yasmin   —people with learning difficulties.

Lesley   But for this group of young people it would be brilliant if it went up to 21, 25.

Jill   I think health visitors are doing a programme with us specifically for the 20 plus, because we're quite aware that there's not much.

Flexibility extended towards groups who were seen as particularly vulnerable, such as young people with learning difficulties, who could access support until they reached 25. Similarly, Penny, who worked with young people with substance abuse issues, could advise them until they were 25. However, the cut-off point for most young people, not just young parents, in terms of accessing support particularly for getting into employment, is 19. As Jill points out, there are few services for young parents aged 20 and over, even though they might be vulnerable and facing the same issues as 18- and 19-year-olds.

McLeod et al. (2006) suggested that a multi-agency approach, with a network of service providers who could signpost and cross-refer between agencies, is the best way of providing support to young mothers. However, at the time of the focus groups, local government funding cuts meant that some services had been reorganised and reduced, or cut completely:

> But it is difficult really, a lot of the funding that was around for courses back into education and supporting people back into work have kind of lost their funding. (Sandra, Seaborough)

This was a situation that had directly impacted on the participants in the Milton focus group, two of whom described how their roles had become much narrower as a result of changes to the way the Connexions service worked. Reorganisation had also affected the staff in Seaborough, with some roles being lost altogether (for example, the young dads' worker) and some being amalgamated.

Aspiration

Returning to education was also linked to aspirations by several participants; whereas some felt that a lack of aspirations had contributed to young people becoming parents, actually being a parent gave them a reason to get better qualifications and possibly a better job. Some participants felt that it was part of their role to raise young people's aspirations, particularly around education:

Rose   I would encourage them to increase their aspirations in life I think. It would be probably nothing to do with pregnancy at all.

Jude   Education, isn't it? Education, yes, what's out there, open their eyes a bit—

Moira   —Yeah—
Jude   —to what else there is in life.
Moira   Yeah, to have a greater self-esteem and bigger aspirations, I think
          that's the biggest thing.
Rose   Yeah.

Arai (2003) found that many of the teenage pregnancy coordinators she interviewed saw their role as a holistic one. This included supporting the young mothers they worked with on a range of issues, rather than having a focus solely on preventing teenage pregnancy, which in itself could cause problems of being seen as 'the enemy' (2003, p. 210). Where services focussed on a single issue, such as education or housing, providers were still keen to take a holistic approach (McLeod et al. 2006). Like many of the participants, Bernie in Carville worked in this way. As well as providing advice and support about education and training, housing, and job seeking, she saw it as part of her role to challenge what she called a 'self-fulfilling prophecy' based on overwhelmingly negative press about young people, and about the area they lived in. She gave several examples of young parents becoming volunteers and some going on to have careers in welfare provision after having been service users, and was proud that the majority of volunteers in the centre where we met were 'home-grown':

> If your expectations of them is that little bit higher, they will rise up to that expectation, do you know what I mean? Might take a bit longer with some than others but they will … they're so used to being told they're rubbish, and it's that self-fulfilling prophecy.

Aspiring to be a Good Parent

As we have seen, the young parents were very keen to position themselves as good parents, and the staff were aware of how many were working very hard at that, but also that for some it could be a challenge. One aspect of doing things differently in terms of aiming to be a good parent related to the poor experiences some young people had had while growing up, particularly for those who had been in care or who had not experienced good relationships with their parents. Some of the interviewees felt that for some young women, a baby would give them a chance to love and be loved that perhaps they had not experienced before:

> It's that cliché I suppose of having somebody to love and to love me, that kind of unconditional love that they've never had as a daughter, where they can be the mother and have it the other way. You know, 'I'm going to be a really good mum and this is going to be my love and my bond that I never had with my mum!' (Ingrid, Norland)

The determination to be a good parent was particularly strong for some young women who had been in care, or who had been adopted, although this could also be a source of stress for them, as they felt that they could not be seen to be failing:

Lynne   I've got a young parent that comes to my group and she was brought up in care, and she had her children young, and she said 'I can't fail at this because I've been brought up in care and I'm a young parent'. So the pressure on her, I mean she works as well, and her partner's got an apprenticeship, so they're both actively in employment, but she said 'I can't fail at it because I was brought up in care and I'm a young parent'. So that massive stress.

Kay   We've got one very similar who again has been through the care system, got three young children, she's only just 20. And she feels the same, wants to have this perfect family where dad lives at home, goes out to work and all of that. But despite being in a really abusive relationship she won't leave because she wants better for her children, that's how she deems it. (Barton)

However, in some cases the staff supporting the young person felt that because they had not experienced a secure and happy family life, they would struggle with parenthood:

> Some of those have gone on to be absolutely some of the best mums I think I've seen. They have really thought consciously, you know, I've heard one girl say, she had a little boy in her arms and she was like 'well

this is the age my mum gave me up and I just can't imagine how she did that!' And she's a fantastic mum, absolutely fantastic, and there's been a few like that, and then you also get the other half that actually can't parent because they haven't got the grounding or the emotional capacity to. (Ingrid, Norland)

For some of the young people, the workers themselves became role models, in some cases because they had been young parents. They then could provide encouragement to young parents as well as proof that it was possible to be a teenage parent and have a professional career:

I was a young parent myself, and it's like 'actually I had a baby when I was 19, I might not be as young as you', but when they say 'oh I want to do your job', well actually you can, you can do that. (Kay, Barton)

Tracy in Barton had also been a teenage mother, and used her experience to demonstrate to the young parents she mentored that it was possible to have a child before the age of 16, and become a professional. Even where the worker was not a parent, they could still provide inspiration. One of the young fathers in Seaborough, who had been disengaged at school and had left with no qualifications, was taking literacy and numeracy courses because he now had an ambition to become a youth worker, saying 'I want to do what [young dads' worker] does'.

One of the advisors who worked with young fathers felt that for many young men, becoming a father was the best thing in their life:

A lot of the lads, it's one of the best things ever happened to them. Things haven't been brilliant throughout their lives, having a child's a kind of whole opportunity, a new identity and step away, if you've been a bit of a wrong 'un, step away from things. And yeah, a lot of lads are quite chuffed. (Sean, Norland)

However, despite the determination of young people to be good parents, there was a great deal of concern about how well they would manage in the economic climate prevailing at the time of the study, with jobs for young people being hard to find in the study locations. Contrary to popular stereotypes, young people did not see life on benefits as an attractive option; many young mothers wanted to return to education or employment once their babies were at school, and many young fathers wanted to support their families. There was a concern that although young people were taking up training opportunities, it would not lead to anything in the long term:

> Everything now is geared around training and qualifications, which is not ensuring they're having jobs at the end of it. It's good for them, you know, and it's good to get them in the training mode, but I think sometimes its false promises because there's still no employment out there. (Bernie, Carville)

The fear amongst people who worked with young parents, felt across England, Scotland and Wales, was that young people would struggle to achieve their aspirations in the current situation. Despite the challenges facing young people and the people providing services to support them, there was a very strong commitment on the part of the interviewees to help young parents succeed:

> With some of the young parents I've met, it's like, well, their parents have survived, they've got through it and they're doing okay, so I can get through it and be okay. But you don't want them to just be okay, do you? You want them to do well and flourish. (Tess, Milton)

A critical factor for many staff was coordination between services, and having the ability to 'signpost' a young parent between services. The advantage of Sure Start Plus had been that it provided a way of bringing different organisations together (Malin and Morrow 2009) and coordinating the support services that could be provided to young parents. Several participants felt that the organisational changes that were taking place at the time of the focus groups meant that such coordination was being lost, with Jon in Barton saying 'I think the silo working mentality is a problem'. He pointed out that although all the agencies would come together if there was a child protection meeting, they would not necessarily know each other's roles. If the holistic approach that Tracy wished for was in operation, it might be possible to prevent individual cases becoming child protection cases:

> My wish list for young parents would be that there was a joined up kind of approach in policy for what things help people, young parents, achieve. So instead of having housing reaching for their targets, health reaching for the targets, that it was a joined up thing that people did together as a team, that holistic work before it gets into the arena of child protection.

Despite the challenges of reorganisation and the consequent danger of fragmentation of services, the individual staff members were committed to providing a holistic service as far as they could. Their experience and accumulated knowledge gained by working in their locations meant that they could work in a coordinated way whether or not formal structures for doing so were in place.

Local Cultures

As Moira, a nurse in Bridgetown said, it felt for many of the staff that there was a culture of acceptance of teenage parenting in their locations, which had histories of people becoming parents at relatively young ages. Many young people would know not only people from their own families—sisters, aunts, mother, grandmother—who perhaps had been a teenage parent, but also friends from school and other people within their communities:

Elaine   A lot of mine seem to be 'oh, well, my sister's pregnant and she's due any day, and my other sister's due and she's got one already', and quite often mum has got a young one as well.

Sandra   I've had a couple of clients that have given birth in the same month as their mum.

Joan   A lot of mine, I would have said it's a case of 'my friend has just had one', and it seems to be they're not out on their own, there's so many others around them having children. (Seaborough)

This meant that young people would not feel unusual or isolated as a young parent, particularly if they were older teenagers. Two of the young mothers in the Norland focus group also felt that it was not unusual in their area to be a young parent:

Fiona   It's the norm round here.
Jane   To be honest I think it's more shocking if you see like a 35-year-old that's pregnant round here than what it is to see someone young.

Clare, a family nurse practitioner in Bridgetown, discussing a programme set up to support young mothers, felt that as the older teens did not label themselves as young mothers, they did not see the programme as something aimed at them:

> I would say there's definitely a different culture here in that young women who are perhaps 18, 19, in particular, are more likely not to engage with the programme because they don't identify themselves as being a young mother … It's a cultural thing, so it's not unusual for us to have grannies in their early thirties and we've got great-grannies who are still in their forties.

In three of the locations, some staff members suggested that there was a tradition of strongly matriarchal families, and that this may have influenced family structures:

> I think there's a very strong female dominant culture in Bridgetown, where we're now maybe third, fourth generation without a male role model in the family, and so I've certainly heard the expression 'we're strong women'. You know, our client, the teenage mother, she's on her own, her mum's on her own, her granny's on her own, so there's also a pattern of not necessarily being in a relationship, a long-term relationship that then continues when you have a baby. (Clare, Bridgetown)

Tracy   I think there is a real kind of strong matriarch legacy that still runs from it being as well like a kind of forces town, the women are quite strong—
Jon   —They were left to run the house, men went to sea for two years, came back, you know.
Kay   Very strong women.

Wendy   Yeah, independent.

Kay   And it can be a very positive thing, extremely positive, but when it goes wrong it's also very powerful, it's very hard to change granny, mum, great-gran's perceptions, you know. (Barton)

This was seen as part of the industrial history and legacy of these locations, with each one having long histories of seafaring, deep-sea fishing, and the armed forces (particularly the Royal Navy) as major employers for men. Chandler found that the Navy wives in her study became accustomed to running a house on their own and making all the domestic decisions (Chandler 1989). Not only are these forms of employment that would lead men to be away at sea for lengthy periods of time, they are also dangerous, with, for example, trawler fishing and merchant seafaring being the two occupations with the highest occupational death rates in the UK (Roberts 2002). Thus, women would not only become accustomed to managing on their own (or with the support of their female relatives) because their partners were away at sea for lengthy periods, they would also be aware that there was a high risk of losing them altogether, and would most likely know other women who had been widowed and were therefore raising children alone. For any woman without a husband, either temporary or permanent, 'life without a husband demands more personal responsibility from women and gives them more power' (Chandler 1991, p. 69).

Futures

All the participants discussed how the past, particularly patterns of employment and patterns of childbearing, had influenced the areas where they worked, areas which had been identified as teenage pregnancy hotspots. But what of the future? As we have seen, the majority of young parents aspire to conventional cultural expectations of getting a job and having a home and family life, and the staff support them and encourage them in those ambitions. However, several participants highlighted the way in which the complexities of the benefit system and the lack of employment opportunities in their area operated in such a way as to make it very difficult for young people to get out of poverty. Bernie explained how some young people had been left without an income because, having got a job and stopped claiming unemployment benefits, they then found themselves working on zero-hours contracts and therefore without a reliable income:

> What happens is if you, say you are claiming benefit, you sign off because you think you've got a full-time job up at the factory. You get there, you might do a full shift the one week, and then it's dribs and drabs everywhere. So if you are a young father, if you have got a family, you haven't got that regular income, you haven't even got the income off the dole then, or whatever you're signing on, you haven't got that money from the government to support you, and you haven't got a full-time wage. So I think it's going to be really hard, really hard.

For some, the possibility of being caught in such a trap meant that taking up work, often low-paid due to having few qualifications, was too risky, and benefits, while not offering a generous income, did at least offer a stable income which they needed to provide for their child:

> Some of the things that I've found with the young parents that I've worked with is it's too much of a risk to take, like with the educational attainment levels that they've got, if they are to go and get a job it's a low-paid job, it's a temporary job, or take up an apprenticeship. So they have to make a choice which is best for themselves and their baby, and that is always going to be the financial stability, and whether that comes from a financially stable job or benefits, I think that's a lot of the time what they decide to do, they're making a decision based on stability I think. (Tracy, Barton)

It was also noted that this particular group were unlikely to have savings or other resources to tide them over in the periods between signing off and being paid, so despite being keen to work, as several participants said, young people were 'stuck between a rock and a hard place':

> People haven't got the savings to be able to say I can live off that, so sometimes it is between a rock and a hard place actually, what do you do? Am I better off as I am? There's lots of young parents out there desperate to go and do something, but actually they need the funds to just get them going. (Kay, Barton)

The challenge for many young parents, then, was how to move into employment that was sufficiently stable for them to be sure they could manage financially, and take the risk of coming off benefits. This study found that, like others (Clarke 2013), the dependency culture does not exist for young people; they do not plan or want to stay on welfare benefits. However, the instability of the employment that is open to them makes it very risky to come off benefits especially as they have few resources to cushion the risk. For many of them, their overarching aim is to provide for their children, and to risk not having any income is one they cannot take.

Conclusions

The many years of experience accumulated by the groups of people interviewed for this chapter enabled participants to have a view on 'what it's like round here' and have provided a perspective on teenage pregnancy and parenting that has rarely been explored to date. In each of the locations, it seemed apparent to the staff that there was an aspect of local culture which meant that for some groups teenage parenting was an accepted norm. However, it was possible to identify particular small areas within their locality where this applied to a greater extent, so although each of the English locations had been identified as a hotspot in the past, the people who worked there could specify parts of their city that had higher rates than other areas. The localities they identified were marked by high levels of social deprivation, high unemployment, and particularly for young people, limited opportunities to find stable, meaningful jobs. Disengagement with the education system was a further characteristic which then itself leads to limited opportunities for employment. Employment patterns were characterised by part-time or zero-hours work which was largely low-skilled and low-paid. It is unsurprising that in this context, many young people feel that they have few opportunities. In contrast to Austerberry and Wiggins (2007), who suggested that Sure Start Plus programmes paid insufficient attention to wider socio-economic contexts in their emphasis on individualistic health and education targets, the staff working in the study locations were very conscious of the context in which their young parents operated. Nevertheless, like the teenage pregnancy coordinator in Chapter 2, who felt that being blamed for failure to hit targets did not acknowledge that she could not influence the wider factors impacting on teenage pregnancy, staff have little influence over poverty and employment in their areas. As a result, like Bernie and the Connexions advisors in Milton, their focus has to be on encouraging young parents to take up educational and training opportunities in the hope that they may be able to find a job, however they feel about the likelihood of them finding meaningful employment.

The other element of local culture identified by participants related to culture within families. The participants identified the same set of reactions amongst many of the families they worked with which the families in this study discussed in Chapter 6; the pregnancy itself may have been a shock and a disappointment, but a baby is welcomed into the family. In a sense, the pregnancy and the baby are regarded as different things; whilst a pregnancy might be unwelcome and unwanted, a baby is neither. Growing up in a culture where family is close and valued, and seeing other people successfully negotiate parenthood at a young age, can, as we saw in Chapter 4, give a young woman a sense that she can manage too.

The overwhelming impression gained by speaking to the people who contributed to this chapter was that they were highly committed to helping and supporting young parents; although they were aware of particular individuals or groups who were more likely to struggle, and knew that there were some who would remain out of reach, they also commended many young parents for doing a good job in difficult circumstances. Their attitudes were non-judgemental, certainly compared to previous generations of people who worked with young mothers, their aim being to help young women keep their babies, not to persuade them to give them up for adoption. In addition, the staff themselves faced challenging circumstances with their jobs being under threat, their roles changing, and their departments being reorganised. Despite facing these difficulties, they were committed to providing stability and continuity for their young clients.

Appendix: Participants in Staff Focus Groups and Interviews

Note: All names are pseudonyms

Name	Role	Location
Sandra	Teenage pregnancy support worker	Seaborough
Elaine	Teenage pregnancy support worker	Seaborough
Joan	Teenage pregnancy support worker	Seaborough
Toni	Teenage parent worker	Norland
Carol	Teenage parent worker	Norland
Sean	Young dads' worker	Norland
Ingrid	Teenage parent worker	Norland
Simon	Team manager (formerly Sure Start Plus coordinator)	Norland
Karen	Community midwife	Milton
Lesley	Advisor, Connexions	Milton
Yasmin	Advisor, Connexions	Milton
Jill	Community development worker (health)	Milton
Penny	Young people's advisor, prevention services	Milton
Tess	Young people's support worker	Milton
Nancy	Young people's support worker	Milton
Lynne	Family social worker	Barton
Kay	Outreach worker, children's centre	Barton
Tracy	Young parent mentor	Barton
Anne	Support worker, children's centre	Barton
Wendy	Outreach worker, children's centre	Barton
Jon	Area manager, children's centres	Barton
Ian	Service commissioning, local authority	Barton
Marion	Community centre support worker	Carville
Bernie	Youth worker	Carville
Clare	Family nurse practitioner	Bridgetown
Moira	Nurse (based in youth drop-in centre)	Bridgetown
Jude	Specialist in Sexual and Reproductive Health services	Bridgetown
Rose	Specialist in Sexual and Reproductive Health services	Bridgetown

References

Arai, L. (2003). Low expectations, sexual attitudes and knowledge: Explaining teenage pregnancy and fertility in English communities. Insights from qualitative research. *The Sociological Review, 51*(2), 199–217.

Austerberry, H., & Wiggins, M. (2007). Taking a pro-choice perspective on promoting inclusion of teenage mothers: Lessons from an evaluation of the Sure Start Plus programme. *Critical Public Health, 17*(1), 3–15.

Brown, S., & Guthrie, K. (2010). Why don't teenagers use contraception? A qualitative interview study. *European Journal of Contraception and Reproductive Health Care, 15*, 197–204.

Chandler, J. (1989). Marriage and the housing careers of naval wives. *The Sociological Review, 37*(2), 253–276.

Chandler, J. (1991). *Women without husbands. An exploration of the margins of marriage.* London: Macmillan.

Clarke, J. (2013). It's not all doom and gloom for teenage mothers – Exploring the factors that contribute to positive outcomes. *International Journal of Adolescence and Youth.* doi:10.1080/02673843.2013.804424.

Coren, E., Barlow, J., & Stewart-Brown, S. (2003). The effectiveness of individual and group-based parenting programmes in improving outcomes for teenage mothers and their children: A systematic review. *Journal of Adolescence, 26*(1), 79–103.

Department for Communities and Local Government. (2012a). *Financial framework for the Troubled Families programme's payment-by-results scheme for local authorities.* London: DCLG.

Department for Communities and Local Government. (2012b). *Listening to troubled families: A report by Louise Casey CBE.* London: DCLG.

Faculty of Sexual and Reproductive Healthcare. (2012). *Drug interactions with hormonal contraception.* Glasgow: FSRH Clinical Effectiveness Unit.

Falk, G., Ivarsson, A. B., & Brynhildsen, J. (2010). Teenagers' struggles with contraceptive use – What improvements can be made? *European Journal of Contraception and Reproductive Health Care, 15*, 271–279.

Ferguson, H., & Gates, P. (2015). Early intervention and holistic, relationship-based practice with fathers: Evidence from the work of the Family Nurse Partnership. *Child and Family Social Work, 20*(1), 96–105.

Forrest, S., Strange, V., Oakley, A., & the RIPPLE study team. (2004). What do young people want from sex education? The results of a needs assessment from a peer-led sex education programme. *Culture, Health and Sexuality, 6*(4), 337–354.

Frost, J. J., Lindberg, L. D., & Finer, L. B. (2012). Young adults' contraceptive knowledge, norms and attitudes: Associations with risk of unintended pregnancy. *Perspectives on Sexual and Reproductive Health, 44*(2), 107–116.

Graham, H., & McDermott, E. (2006). Qualitative research and the evidence base of policy: Insights from studies of teenage mothers in the UK. *Journal of Social Policy, 35*(1), 21–37.

Gregson, J. (2009). *The culture of teenage mothers*. New York: SUNY Press.

Jewell, D., Tacchi, J., & Donovan, J. (2000). Teenage pregnancy: Whose problem is it? *Family Practice, 17*(6), 522–528.

Joseph, K. (1974). Speech at the Grand Hotel, Birmingham, UK, 19th October 1974. Retrieved from http://www.margaretthatcher.org/archive/displaydocument.asp?docid=101830

Kelly, D. (2000). *Pregnant with meaning: Teen mothers and the politics of inclusive schooling*. New York: Peter Lang Publishing.

Kidger, J. (2004). Including young mothers: Limitations to New Labour's strategy for supporting teenage parents. *Critical Social Policy, 24*(3), 291–311.

Kirkman, M., Harrison, M., Hillier, L., & Pyett, P. (2001). 'I know I'm doing a good job': Canonical and autobiographical narratives of teenage mothers. *Culture, Health and Sexuality, 3*(3), 279–294.

Luttrell, W. (2003). *Pregnant bodies, fertile minds: Gender, race and the schooling of pregnant teens*. New York: Routledge.

Malin, N., & Morrow, G. (2009). Evaluating the role of the Sure Start Plus Adviser in providing integrated support for pregnant teenagers and young parents. *Health and Social Care in the Community, 17*(5), 495–503.

McLeod, A., Baker, D., & Black, M. (2006). Investigating the nature of formal social support provision for young mothers in a city in the North West of England. *Health and Social Care in the Community, 14*(6), 453–464.

Moran, P., Ghate, D., & van der Merwe, A. (2004). *What works in parenting support? A review of the international evidence*. London: DfES.

Murray, C. (1990). *The emerging British underclass*. London: IEA.

Pratt, R., Stephenson, J., & Mann, S. (2014). What influences contraceptive behaviour in women who experience unintended pregnancy? A systematic review of qualitative research. *Journal of Obstetrics and Gynaecology, 34*, 693–699.

Roberts, S. (2002). Hazardous occupations in Great Britain. *The Lancet, 360*(9332), 543–544.

Salihi, S., Brown, D. W., Melrose, E., & Merchant, S. (2002). Revisiting a pilot survey involving contraception and teenage pregnancy in Ayrshire and Arran. *Journal of Family Planning and Reproductive Health Care, 28*(1), 37–38.

Scottish Parliament. (2013). Fifth report, 2013 (Session 4): Report on inquiry into teenage pregnancy, HC/S4/13/R5. Edinburgh: Scottish Government.

Shoveller, J., Chabot, C., Johnson, J. L., & Prkachin, K. (2011). 'Ageing out': When policy and social orders intrude on the 'disordered' realities of young mothers. *Youth and Society, 43*(4), 1355–1380.

Smith, S., & Ratcliffe, A. (2009). Women's education and childbearing: A growing divide. In J. Stillwell, E. Coast, & D. Kneale (Eds.), *Fertility, living arrangements, care and mobility. Understanding population trends and processes, vol. 1*. London: Springer.

Vincent, K., & Thomson, P. (2010). 'Slappers like you don't belong in this school': The educational inclusion/exclusion of pregnant schoolgirls. *International Journal of Inclusive Education, 14*(4), 371–385.

Yardley, E. (2009). Teenage mothers' experiences of formal support services. *Journal of Social Policy, 38*(2), 241–257.

8

'It's Mad How Much You Grow up': The Future for Young Parents and Their Children

Becoming a mother for the first time, for most women and of whatever age, means taking on a new role, adopting a new identity, and sometimes leaving a previous way of life behind. To become a mother as a teenager is to take on an adult role at a time when a young woman may be deciding what to 'be', and is still developing and shaping her identity. Indeed, one of the catchy sound bites used by politicians about teenage parents that specifically focusses on their age and immaturity is that they are 'children having children', suggesting that they are growing up and taking on adult roles too soon. In this chapter, I explore how the young people feel about growing up and becoming parents, what they want for their children, and how they see their future. As their parents had talked about wanting better for their teenagers, so the teenagers talked about how they would encourage their children to do better than they had; I will discuss this in the context of the meaning of parenthood to the young people, and in particular how this sits within an understanding of what it means to be a good mother or father, and to do a good job of raising children of whom they can be proud, and who will, they hope, be proud of them. Using a framework of youth transitions, particularly relating to class and

© The Editor(s) (if applicable) and The Author(s) 2016
S. Brown, *Teenage Pregnancy, Parenting and Intergenerational Relations*,
DOI 10.1057/978-1-137-49539-6_8

gender, will facilitate a discussion of whether, and how, young people sit within traditional patterns of transitions to adulthood. The 'Inventing Adulthoods' study, by a team led by Rachel Thomson at South Bank University, London, is a longitudinal study with young people taking place over five years at various UK locations, looking at how and when young people make transitions to adulthood, and how that is changing. Several papers from the study have been useful in formulating ideas about transitions, class and gender for this chapter.

Transition to Adulthood

Thomson and Holland (2002) discuss the extent to which relationships between genders are changing, particularly in terms of women's lives and expectations. In their view, while the individualisation theories put forward by Beck (1992) and Beck and Beck-Gernscheim (1995) and the theories of detraditionalisation suggested by Heelas et al. (1996) go some way to explaining how change is happening, they do not fully explain the complexities of change, particularly for young women. Other writers (MacDonald et al. 2005; Furlong and Cartmel 2007) argue that although change in young people's lives may have become more complex, varied and extended, the concept of youth transitions itself remains valuable, particularly in examining how young people's lives remain influenced by their original position in the class structure. Walkerdine et al. (2001) also discuss social class as a factor, and see young women as a '"subject" of modern neo-liberalism' (Thomson and Holland 2002, p. 338), particularly in terms of self-regulation and self-invention, suggesting that 'the most seductive aspect of self-invention of all lies in the possibility of the working class remaking itself as middle class' (Walkerdine et al. 2001, p. 21). The issues of self-regulation and self-invention are particularly salient for young women who become mothers, largely because by becoming mothers at a point that society deems too young, they have breached the neo-liberal ideal both by failing to regulate themselves (by becoming pregnant) and by failing to reinvent themselves in the model of a neo-liberal discourse of success, whereby success comes through education and labour market participation (McRobbie 2009); using Walkerdine's framing, they have failed to reinvent themselves as middle class.

Furthermore, Thomson and Holland argue that although Beck's distinction between 'normal' and 'choice' biographies has been used to explain increasingly fragmented routes for young people to transition to adulthood, particularly a 'gender specific normal biography' (Du Bois-Reymond 1998, p. 66) and a 'non-gender specific choice biography', it is overly simplistic. They suggest that Du Bois-Reymond's argument that gender is becoming much less of a determining influence pays insufficient attention to the continuing existence of traditional pathways which operate very differently for young men and young women, particularly in choices around career and family. Nilsen and Brannen's (2002) analysis is more convincing as they emphasise 'the continuing significance of structural inequalities which provide the parameters within which individual choices are made' (Thomson and Holland 2002, p. 338). While Nilsen and Brannen suggest that inequalities in available resources influence the choices that young people think they have, I would suggest that the currently widening inequalities in the UK may narrow the range of choices that young people think are open to them. Thomson and Holland found that the majority of young people in their study, when asked to think about their future life path, followed a normative model of career, marriage and family by the age of 35, and suggest that they are 'constrained by a resilient model of adulthood anchored in heteronormative notions of settling down' (2002, p. 348). They argue that youth transitions are fluid, but that they remain structured by class and gender as well as by race and locality.

Transition to adulthood is now characterised by uncertainty, with many traditional routes no longer existing, although this varies by class (Thomson et al. 2004). Young people travel at different rates along different routes (Thomson et al. 2002), with the speed and timing of transition to adulthood also varying by class, with an extension of adolescence particularly for middle-class young people, who continue in full-time education into their twenties, and may not establish their own home until their late twenties. As a result, 'the meanings of adulthood are created within particular classed and gendered cultures' (Thomson et al. 2004, p. 219) which results in contested meaning around many defining experiences, motherhood being a significant example (Thomson 2000). Thomson et al. (2002) used the concept of a 'critical moment' to describe how young people's biographies relate to social processes; I will now go on to explore how the critical moment of parenthood acts as a social process of growing up, and how parenthood can be 'the first act of adulthood' (Thomson et al. 2011, p. 2).

Becoming Grown up

Several of the young people talked about growing up as something that has to happen as a result of becoming a parent:

> It's mental how much you grow up when you have kids. You've got to grow up, you've got to be responsible, and it's mad. (Megan)

In other words, becoming a parent propels an individual along the transitional route and into adulthood. Naomi was clear that she was no longer the same teenage self she had been at the point at which she became pregnant:

> I was still only just kind of just turned a teenager and was going out to party, if you like, and then it was all over (laughs).

She talks as if the life of a carefree teenager has ended for her almost before it began, but that this was not a problem because she barely knew that life anyway:

> I suppose what you don't know, you don't miss, so it didn't bother me that way.

In the second interview with Naomi, when her partner Jamie also took part, they talked about how 'having a baby grows you up a lot' (Naomi) but this was a good thing because:

Naomi   I think for us it's for the better because it's made us have broad shoulders, so like if we didn't have Jordan, anything could have happened, do you know what I mean? Like a lot of people drop out of college—

Jamie   —You get more drive.

Naomi   Yeah, it definitely does, it makes you more driven.

Having a baby is both the process that makes a teenager into an adult, and a reason to become more adult-like, in terms of being driven, and in Jamie's case, wanting to make sure he still manages to stick to his plan of going to university and then either becoming a teacher or eventually starting his own business. They also talked about getting married both as something they wanted for themselves but also as a signifier to others of their maturity:

Naomi   We want to get married as well because, it's going to be really sloppy this, on your recording, but I couldn't feel for anyone else and I don't think he could—or he better not! (Laughing)

Jamie   Like as well, if you say 'me and my girlfriend have got a baby', it sounds more childish whereas if I say 'me and my fiancée' or 'my partner', you sound more mature and steady, and I think it shows that we are serious about it, that we are stable.

Naomi   But then it's not just for everyone else's benefit so anyone else thinks that we're stable, it's for ourselves.

We have already seen in Chapter 5 how for many young people, the transition to parenthood can be a significant turning point in their lives, making some, like Katy, think about what they want in life and providing an incentive to achieve it:

> If I hadn't had Josh I wouldn't have gone to TPU, I wouldn't have gone on any of my courses … I'd've ended up just being on dole probably and ending up with jobs that I don't like, whereas now I'm teaching and I get to support people … I have like a lot of people around me now who are proud of me for what I have done and if I hadn't have done that, I'd have ended up just working in my dad's shop in the end because he would have had enough of me, he'd have just said 'get to work' and that'll be it … my life would be crap to be fair (laughs).

For others, such as Steve and Ella, it meant a physical turning point as well as an emotional one, moving house with their son to what they felt was a nicer area, and getting away from Steve's old associates, with whom he had got into trouble. Looking back at his old self from the vantage point of fatherhood and a relationship, he says:

> I was dead childish, I was dead immature, as soon as I found out I was having him, that's it, I changed.

Edin and Kefalas (2005) discuss how for many women in their study, motherhood was perceived as having saved them, their baby bringing 'the purpose, the validation, the companionship and the order' (2005, p. 10) that was lacking in their lives. In this way, mothering takes primacy in their lives as a source of identity and meaning as part of a redemptive process. A similar redemption process seems to operate for young men, particularly those, like Steve, who have previously been engaged in criminal activities and been to prison. Research on why young people stop offending suggests that access to material opportunities, such as education and employment, and opportunities to establish social bonds such as having a stable family life, play a role. MacDonald (2006) and MacDonald and Shildrick (2007) show that an important aspect of this transition for an individual is being able to move away from the self-image of being an offender, and assume a better identity, as Steve does here, where he moves from a condemnation script to a redemption script (Maruna 2001). There is plenty of evidence that young women re-evaluate their lives and reduce risky behaviour as part of the transition to motherhood (SmithBattle 2007), and it appears that fatherhood can perform the same role for young men.

Hosie (2007) reviews some of the literature on social exclusion and pregnancy from the point of view of the impact of pregnancy on education and says that 'pregnancy during teenage years is predominantly viewed as a negative end point in the trajectory of a young woman's life' (2007, p. 334). Although she concludes that the young women in her study could have a positive outcome to their pregnancy in terms of re-engagement with education, the idea of pregnancy being an end point in a life trajectory is left unexamined. It might be suggested that the end point refers to the end of adolescence, and as Naomi alludes to above, the end of teenage fun when it has barely begun. Some young women are very conscious that becoming a mother necessitates a change in behaviour;

although Becky, eight months pregnant at the time of the focus group, says she had no choice but to be responsible now, her pregnancy was planned and she positioned herself as someone who was mature and experienced enough to make that decision:

> I have changed responsibly because you have to, you don't have a choice when you see them two pink lines, it's time to stop partying, put the alcoholic beverage down and pick up the bottles of milk.

Being a Good Mum

As well as taking on an identity as a mother, young women strive to be seen as good mothers. Rolfe (2008) shows how young women construct their identities as good mothers, despite dominant ideas about mothering being based on white middle-class norms. Women in her study were marginalised not only economically, but also discursively as not being 'good' mothers because they did not fit the norms of good motherhood. However, they did not position themselves as marginalised. Teenage mothers are aware of their position as a member of a stigmatised group (Rolfe 2008; Yardley 2009), but being able to claim to be a good mother enables them to distinguish themselves from this narrative (McDermott and Graham 2005; Romagnoli and Wall 2012), by adopting what Kirkman et al. (2001) call a 'consoling plot'. In a similar way to young mothers in other studies (for example Phoenix 1991; Mitchell and Green 2002), the young women in my study were keen to present themselves as 'good' mothers who are responsible and caring. They talked about 'doing the best for your child' in terms of being present, providing a loving and caring atmosphere, and putting their children first:

Jane   A good mum is someone who looks after their kids, and puts their kids first no matter what.

Fiona   Yeah, I think you're a good mum if, when you have your kids, what you enjoy changes instantly when you have them. Like I don't like going out drinking now or partying or anything like what I used to like.

Ingrid	But are you a bad mum if you still do?
Fiona	If you do it every day.
Steph	Putting your kids' needs first above your needs, above your wants, above everything, it's your kids' needs.

Having said that 'it's really hard to define being a good mum', Nikki went on to describe some of the qualities a good mother would have:

> It's all different things, isn't it? Obviously being there for your kids, putting them first. Just bring your kids up, put them first, make sure they're polite and things like that and do everything you can for your kids I suppose, protecting them and things like that. I don't know, there's so many things, isn't there, to being a good mum.

Most of the young parents focussed on caring qualities such as 'being there', rather than having resources in terms of money and consumer goods. The only person to mention material goods specifically was Megan, in the context of provision of clothes and food, as one aspect of how a mother would know she was doing a good job:

> As long as the kids are provided for, then you haven't got nothing to worry about. As long as you know you've got the help you need if you need it, and as long as you know you've got the money to look after them and as long as they're clothed, fed, in school, good education, that's all they need.

Although the issue of money and finances arose in several interviews and focus groups, it was in the sense of making sure there was enough to get by, as Megan suggests, having enough to feed and clothe the children and pay for essentials such as household bills. For many parents the most important resources were effort and time:

Jackie	Just do everything you can to just make sure that they're happy and healthy, even if it's like the hardest thing that you've ever had to do, which it is, especially when you've got like a demanding child, if it's the hardest thing that you've ever had to do, and you will ever have to do, you've just got to make sure that they don't know that it's hard.

Jane   Just spend time with them, do anything, talk to them, nursery rhymes, painting, playing, bonding.

Having time also connected with affection; love and cuddles were important, and several parents talked about the 'best bits' of time with their children being when they had time in the morning or the evening for cuddling and playing:

Steve   The smiles and the laughs, I love the giggles, I love his giggles.
Ella   Because he knows you're still there.
Steve   Yeah, and now he's started saying da da, I love that.
Mel   I think mine are cuddles, in the morning. When they first wake you up.
Steve   Yeah.
Ella   Mmm.

The same applied for Becky and Sharon who were yet to become mothers:

Becky   Stability, routine and love.
Sharon   Cuddles.
Jenny   She was real serious, stability! (laughs)

Jenny teases Becky about being serious, but as Becky was at that point eight months pregnant, living in a hostel and hoping that she and her partner Carl would manage to rent a house before the baby was born, her wish for stability is unsurprising.

Being a Good Dad

Young fathers also want to construct an identity as a good father. Tuffin et al. (2010) show how the stereotypes that pathologise teenage parents as a whole position young men as uncaring, selfish and callous. However, the young men in their study, based in New Zealand, wanted to be good fathers, and constructed a discourse of responsibility as a key part of this. For them, the breadwinner role whereby they would provide for their family and look after them was a core aspect of being a good father. Carl, in one of the focus groups in Seaborough, said it was important to provide for his family; he had a job, and although he said there were possibilities for promotion in the company where he worked, he said that was not the sort of person he was, as he just wanted to know he was earning enough to provide for his family:

> Food on the table and a nice house. Leave all the bills and whatnot to her.

He would leave the running of the house ('the bills and whatnot') to Becky, who had already set out to position herself as someone who was responsible and knew how to manage. Steve and Ella also had a traditionally gendered idea of their roles as parents:

Steve   I'm looking for work; she's going to be in.
Ella   I want to stay at home.
Steve   She's going to be a stay-at-home housewife.
Ella   Yeah, until he's in full-time school.

Deslauriers (2011) also found that young men constructed an identity as a father based on a willingness to take on responsibility and on working to meet the needs of their child. For the Seaborough young men, being a good dad encompassed a range of activities, including traditional household tasks, but with a strong focus for Carl and Dave here on education:

SB   One of you is a dad, one of you is going to be a dad. How would you describe what a good dad is?
Jenny   A lot of patience (everyone laughs).
Carl   Loads of things really.
Dave   Being supportive.
Carl   Yeah. First and foremost, providing things. Education. Just doing dad things, the simplest things, such as gardening (everyone laughs). It is, isn't it though, really?
Dave   Good tea making!
Carl   The most simplest things have the biggest effect.
SB   When you say education do you mean—

Carl   Sitting down with your kids and doing their maths homework with them, even though I'm not good at it.

Becky   Which he can do because I can't do maths! I'm good at English which is usually the case, isn't it, if you're good at English you're bad at maths.

Sharon   Which one of you is doing the birds and the bees talk? I've told my boyfriend he's doing it!

Carl   If it's a boy I'll do it, otherwise she can, I'm not dealing with all those hormones! (everyone laughs)

None of this group were in education at this point; Sharon (four months pregnant) and Carl were both working, Dave was unemployed and looking for work, Jenny was at home with her eight-week-old baby (and planning to return to college in due course), and Becky was eight months pregnant. From the laughter at Carl's suggestion that 'doing dad things' included gardening, the discussion switched quickly to the role of homework; education meant school and 'common sense', not university and post-compulsory education:

SB   So in terms of education, supporting them at school?

Dave   Yeah.

Carl   Yeah.

Jenny   Yeah. Making sure they do their homework.

Dave   I think it's good to have a good education, I mean not necessarily university and stuff but—

Jenny   —general knowledge and you know—

Dave   —teach them common sense. I think, in a way, not making it always as if the world's perfect, but not saying that everything goes wrong.

Jenny   But making sure that they understand that it's difficult. Make sure that they know that it's good to struggle sometimes because you learn from it.

The issue of whether or not a parent should let their children know that they had struggled was one where there were some differences in opinion. Whereas Jenny and Dave felt it was good for children to know that life could sometimes be a struggle, like Jackie above, Jane felt that one way of being a good mum was for her children not to realise that it had been hard for her:

Ingrid   So how would you feel if Daisy came home, how old were you? Sixteen when you were pregnant with Daisy, if she came home at 16, and said 'Mum, I'm pregnant'?

Jane   I'd sort of feel like I've not shown her the way, if you know what I mean, but I'd also feel like she mustn't have seen how hard it was for me, which makes me feel like a good mum, because I've not shown her how hard it is.

Ingrid   That's what we were saying this morning, about girls that are young mums, whose mums have been young mums, they see their mums as doing a really good job anyway so why is it an issue?

Jane   Yeah, but then I'm also going to say to her when she's old enough to understand, it was hard, and it would be nice for you to be able to live your life. But I wouldn't be devastated or anything like that, it's not what I want for her but it's her life, she can choose to live it the way she wants to.

Like Paula earlier, Jane plans to tell Daisy that life as a teenage mother is hard, and hopes that she waits until she is older to become a mother, but she also hopes that Daisy will not realise how hard it has been for her.

Don't be Like Me: Education and the Future

As we saw earlier, it is common for parents to say they want better for their children, and one aspect of this is saying 'don't be like me', although that then introduces the dilemma of 'did I ruin your life?' Naomi and Jamie are well aware of this dilemma and it is part of what spurs them to be as driven and ambitious as they are. Here, on the first occasion I met her, Naomi explains that she is happy that Jamie has managed to stay on at sixth form college and stick to his plan to go to university:

I'm glad he's staying on with everything and not getting knocked off course, so that's good, because when you are a teenage mum, a pregnant teenager, people just tend to judge you and think 'oh, you are going to be on dole all your life, you are not even going to try', but me and my boyfriend had thought, 'well, we are not going to let him down', we want him to grow up and think 'well, at least they tried for me', you know? Rather than just giving up and just dropping out of everything. I didn't want him to like feel the pressure, like 'oh well I'm the one that ruined your life then', you know, when he gets older. So we've carried on for him.

Four months later, Jamie explained why it was important for him to carry on with his education:

Jamie   I think just like 20 years down the line, I want to be a teacher, so getting the degree would let me do that when I wanted.

Naomi   Yeah, he plans ahead for quite a while quite a lot.

Jamie   This time last year I wouldn't have been able to do it, but it's only because he's made me more driven, and like, I have to think about these things.

Naomi   So more sensible as well.

Jamie   Because if I think, like my parents offered to help me out with university and stuff, and I want to be in the situation where I can do that with my family, so that's going to be happening 20 years down the line. I need to be in the situation where I can do it.

In one way, Naomi and Jamie were an unusual couple, as far as the study was concerned, in that they had both planned to go to university. Although Naomi had put her plans to be a teacher to one side, Jamie, with her support, had stuck to his original ambitions. It had not been straightforward for him; he was attending a sixth form college in Seaborough when his son Jordan was born, and had taken time off to be at home with Naomi. He had passed his AS exams, but despite this, had been asked not to return to college for the second year of A level studies because of his attendance record. His explanation, that he had become a father and needed time at home, was not sufficient, and he had been obliged to leave. His response had been to approach another sixth form college in the city and explain his situation, and he had been accepted there for the final year of his pre-university studies. As we saw earlier, there is research about the impact of pregnancy on girls' education in the UK (Hosie 2007; Vincent and Thomson 2010) and in the USA (Kelly 2000; Luttrell 2003) but the impact on young men's education of their girlfriend being pregnant and them becoming a young father has been overlooked.

Links between a lack of engagement with school and teenage pregnancy are well established (SEU 1999; Hosie 2007; Vincent and Thomson 2010) and as we saw in Chapter 7, people who work with young parents know that in the locations where the study took place, there is a relationship between non-attendance at school and teenage pregnancy. The focus group discussion above showed how the young parents (Jenny and Dave) and parents-to-be (Becky and Carl, Sharon) prioritised supporting their children's education as something a good dad would do, and as Clarke (2013) found, young parents have a high level of commitment to and high aspirations for their children. For some young parents, education came within the 'wanting better' discourse that parents of all generations engaged with, where it meant 'don't be like me' as far as school was concerned:

> I want Elen to be the opposite of me. I want her to finish school, do her GCSEs, have a nice job, meet someone, make a family after you've lived your life. I want her and Aled to be like that, because I've always wished that. Sometimes I've sat and thought what would you be doing now if you didn't have kids? And I'm just like I don't know, because I've never known what I wanted to do when I was younger. (Megan)

Looking to her future, Amy, who had been truanting from school since her early teens and at the time of her interview was living in foster care after passing through the criminal justice system, said:

> I'd like to have a good—be good and have a good life and he don't leave school and stuff like that. I'd tell him to stick with school because I wasn't good at it.

In saying she wants to 'be good', having just explained that she had a criminal record by the time she had her son, it appears that Amy may be turning towards a redemption script in wanting to change her life now she is a mother.

As well as wanting to be good parents and encourage their children to work at school and get an education, many of the young people aspired to completing their education themselves. As we saw earlier, Jamie plans to go to university, and one of the young mothers in the Seaborough focus group, Faye, was at university. She had her baby after finishing her A levels, and had taken a year out and then taken up her university place. However, Jamie and Faye were unusual in aiming to have a degree-level education. Patti, in Milton, said she would like to get a degree, but she had left school before completing her A levels and was not attending college, so, like Katy, university seemed to be something she might like to do, rather than putting plans in place to achieve it. It was much more common amongst the study participants to be studying for NVQs; some had been at college when they found out they were pregnant, and planned to return once the baby was born, such as Debbie, who was studying childcare.

Both Haley and Naomi had been at school when they found they were pregnant. As we saw earlier, Naomi left school because of the bullying she had experienced due to her pregnancy. By the time of her second interview, she had started a college course which was very different to her original ambition, but which she was enjoying:

> I didn't want to drop out completely so I just changed courses to a two-day course on hairdressing, which turns out I do want to carry on with that now, just a backup in case, because I just didn't want to drop out, do you know what I mean? But I did want to be an English specialist teacher.

Haley had left sixth form because she had been ill during her pregnancy; finding full-time education too much, she had attended the 'schoolgirl mums' unit prior to her son being born, and by the time he was six months old was attending full-time and taking as many courses as she could manage, mostly around childcare and health and social care:

I haven't decided what I want to do yet. I just know that if I do so many [courses] I'll have a choice. So I think teaching assistant is going to end up being the way I'm going to go. It's the one I enjoy the most because I get to spend a lot of time with bairns but I don't know, it depends. Depends how other things take me. If I do my health and social I'll be able to go and work in care homes and stuff, with elderly and stuff like that, works either way.

Far from being the end point of an educational trajectory, which Hosie (2007) suggested is a common way of regarding a teenage pregnancy, for the young women in this study pregnancy caused some to pause and then resume education, much as older women would take maternity leave in a career, or for others was an incentive to re-engage with education. However, as Vincent and Thomson (2010, p. 382) argue, 'the consequences of their school experiences are thus more than simply social exclusion but are also economic and political' (2010, p. 382) because of the types of courses that the young women take, and the jobs that these will lead to, which are likely to be low-paid, and few opportunities for advancement. Naomi is an example of this, leaving her teaching ambitions to one side and changing to hairdressing. However, an alternative interpretation is that some occupations, such as hairdressing and beauty, can provide some flexibility and freedom which a more conventional job might not; if, for example, it is possible to work freelance as a hairdresser doing home visits, childcare might be easier to manage than, say, for a school teacher.

None of the young men talked about returning to education; some were working (such as Carl) but those who were not working wanted to find a job, although they described how difficult it was, not least because there were large numbers of applicants for any jobs advertised. As we saw in Chapter 3, the areas where the focus groups were held tended to have a high ratio of applicants for jobs, and higher than the national average levels of youth unemployment:

Steve   There's all these people, about 5,000 people applying for one job or five jobs. Something in a pub, like The Bowling Green, they were looking for 200 staff, I think it was, 15,000 people applied for 200 jobs, and they weren't even from here, they were from all over, from like [towns 20 and 30 miles away] and everywhere, so it's getting harder to find a job. Even when the steelworks were open and everything it was dead easy, just go in and say 'I've got no experience but I'm a quick learner', so I could get a job straightaway, but it's getting more down now.

Ella   A lot of it's about who you know now as well. If you know someone who works there, they can say 'he is actually a hard worker', and you're more likely to get it.

Shildrick et al. (2012) talk about the low-pay/no-pay cycle as being characteristic of young people's working patterns as they move between spells of unemployment and low-paid, insecure jobs, and this 'churn' was being experienced by several of the young men, including Dave in Seaborough, Mark in Norland and Steve in Milton:

Steve   I had a job, I had a full-time job and everything; I was working 12-hour shifts six days a week. And I lost my job just before we had him, didn't I?

Ella   Just before he was born.

Steve   I got made redundant so I'm trying every single option I can to try and get a job, I've applied for loads of different jobs, I'm just not getting anywhere at the moment.

Mark had also had a job for four months before being made redundant, and although he had been on a number of training schemes, had not yet found another job. Despite their experiences, all the young men were committed to finding work. MacDonald et al. describe this as a 'hyperconventional attitude to work' whereby trying to get any kind of job was 'the driving force behind most youth transitions' (2005, p. 882) amongst the young people in their working-class area of Teesside.

Aspiration and Social Mobility

Writing in 2003, Thomson et al. suggested that opportunities for social mobility were fewer then than for the past 20 years, despite the expansion of higher and further education in the UK. Dorling has argued more recently that social destiny is more than ever determined by where and to whom one is born, suggesting that social mobility is even less likely now, in 2015, than 12 years ago (Dorling 2015). The expansion of higher education does not seem to have had much impact on the young people in this study; as we have seen, only one was at university and very few aspired to go. Despite evidence that social mobility is decreasing in the UK (McNight 2015; Ashley et al. 2015), politicians talk about it as desirable and achievable for all, if only individuals could realise that it was possible: the UK Prime Minister, David Cameron, speaking in November 2013, for example, said that social mobility was being held back because people outside the middle classes did not have high aspirations, saying that it was necessary to 'win people over and raise their aspirations and get them to get all the way to the top' (Mason and Wintour 2013). Mentioning the judiciary, politics and journalism as examples, Cameron seems unaware that those are three of the more difficult occupations to access for young people from working-class backgrounds without resources or contacts. However, the main issue with the argument is not about specific occupations, but about the individualising of aspiration: not 'getting to the top' becomes a failure of individual ambition, with structural inequalities and disadvantage going unaddressed. Thomson et al. (2003) suggest that young people in Britain had embraced an individualistic 'can do' philosophy which fitted in with the New Labour discourse of social improvement and the policy emphasis on reducing social exclusion, which was discussed in Chapter 2. A further issue with the aspiration agenda which is rarely questioned relates to what counts as an acceptable aspiration; for politicians, it almost always seems to equate to getting a university education and having a highly paid career. In other words, as Walkerdine et al. (2001) suggest, young people from working-class backgrounds must reinvent themselves as middle class. However, when talking about their desires and hopes for the future, the young parents wanted a job but talked much more about what they wanted for themselves and their children in terms of happiness, stability and security; a life in which a job played a part but was not the defining factor of success. Asked where they would like to see themselves in two years' time, the replies were quite consistent in the themes that they contained:

Settled in my own home with Riley. But hopefully I'm in a stable job and everything, enough to provide for me and him. (Haley)

I'll hopefully have my own business up and running, definitely working, if not that, just definitely working. Louise to be in school and really settled and popular, like hard-working at school. (Nikki)

Steve   I want to be in a full-time job again.

Ella   I just want to be with Steve and Scott in two years.

Steve   Hopefully be married as well.

Ella   I'm not even bothered if we're married or not, I just still want to be with him. I want to be lucky enough to be able to stay with you, and that's the truth. Jobs, money, anything else I don't care, as long as he's happy and I've still got the love, that's it.

Patti   Oh, that was dead sweet, weren't it!

Despite Patti's teasing of Ella for being 'sweet', participants were open in talking about their love for each other, and all of those who took part as couples talked about having a future together with their children, whether or not that included marriage. Patti herself was engaged, but said she would not get married:

Patti   Yeah, I'm all for people being happy but being married is a whole different kettle of fish.

Mel   Even though you're engaged?

Patti   Yeah, I'm engaged, but I'm very unlikely to ever get married. It just makes things more complicated when you've got to explain to your kids we're having a divorce and everything's taking three times as long because we've got to sign off everything and we've got to share everything.

Although Patti might seem cynical in talking about divorce, in this respect her attitude is similar to the women in Edin and Kefalas' study (2005), who, they suggested, value marriage so highly that they would not marry the fathers of their children until they were sure the men were worthy of it, and the marriage would work.

As well as knowing what they wanted, the young people were clear about what they did not want, or plan to do:

> We don't want to be on the dole all our lives, we want to actually do it ourselves, be able to say 'I bought this house myself' and I'm doing it all off my own back, that's why we're still trying hard. Even though it's a lot harder for us. (Naomi)

They saw themselves as needing benefits temporarily until they were able to get a job, or to help while they completed college courses which they saw as leading to better jobs in the future.

The current policy approach, insofar as it addresses a social exclusion agenda without actually calling it that, is that aspirations are lower in more deprived areas and that this is the problem. However, recent research (Baars 2014) suggests that young people living in deprived areas adopt particular forms of aspiration which involve lower levels of skills and training, and not that they have no aspirations. A further issue is how young people are expected to achieve their high aspirations, and this is often based on an assumption that they will be geographically mobile, and be able and willing to abandon their attachment to place and family (Allen and Hollingworth 2013). Unless they have resources and networks to support them, this is hard enough for any young person; for young parents who may be dependent on a geographically close family and wider social networks for being able to manage day-to-day life, it is near impossible.

Walkerdine et al. (2001) suggest that middle-class families define success in relation to achievement, whether academic or professional, whereas working-class families define it in relation to happiness. In policy approaches, middle-class norms are privileged both in terms of what is an acceptable aspiration and how it should be achieved. However, this is a limited view of success in life, where happiness and being a good parent are not prioritised. Thomson et al. (2003) suggest that as social mobility is so limited, more consideration should be given to incorporating happiness as a component of social exclusion.

Conclusions

The concept of transition has been widely critiqued, not least by some of the writers I considered at the beginning of this chapter, who prefer theories that focus on individualisation (Beck 1992; Beck and Beck-Gernscheim 1995; Du Bois-Reymond 1998). However, although transitions from adolescence to adulthood are more fragmented, variable and, for some young people, extended than in the past, the concept of transition is still useful in terms of exploring processes of becoming adult. It is particularly useful alongside the concept of the 'critical moment' in examining how one such critical moment—becoming a parent—influences 'growing up', and itself is influenced by class and gender.

For most young people, certainly the ones who took part in this study, becoming a parent meant becoming an adult. Many of them had become householders, though few were home-owners, and those who remained living with their parents planned to have their own home as soon as it was practical. All of them were the primary carers for their children, and although the children's grandparents (and other family members) helped with childcare, both groups were aware of the fine line between helping and taking over. Indeed, some had moved into their own homes in order to become a mother their own way, and not have the mothering role taken over by the baby's grandmother. As part of the transition to adulthood, motherhood becomes a critical moment at which point a young woman can carve out a valued identity for herself as a mother and a responsible adult. The concept of responsibility came through in many interviews, and young people were keen to present themselves as in this light, parenthood being both a responsible choice, and a site where responsibility could be demonstrated. The paths young people take appear to be clearly gendered; young men like Steve and Carl follow a traditional breadwinner script in wanting to work so they can provide for their families. Within the wider family, although there might be concern about the timing, motherhood itself is valued because it brings the next generation into the family, and allows the older generation to make their own transition to grandparenthood, something they may have been looking forward to, and a role they expect to enjoy.

The young people in this study are rooted in place and family, and although this may limit their opportunities they still have aspirations—just maybe not to be a barrister.

References

Allen, K., & Hollingworth, S. (2013). 'Sticky subjects' or 'cosmopolitan creatives'? Social class, place and urban young people's aspirations for work in the knowledge economy. *Urban Studies, 50*(3), 499–517.

Ashley, L., Duberley, J., Sommerlad, H., & Scholarios, D. (2015). *A qualitative evaluation of non-educational barriers to the elite professions.* London: Social Mobility and Child Poverty Commission.

Baars, S. (2014). *Place, space and imagined futures: How young people's occupational aspirations are shaped by the areas they live in.* Ph.D. thesis. University of Manchester, Faculty of Humanities.

Beck, U. (1992). *Risk Society: Towards a new modernity.* London: Sage.

Beck, U., & Beck-Gernsheim, E. (1995). *The normal chaos of love.* Cambridge: Polity Press.

Clarke, J. (2013). It's not all doom and gloom for teenage mothers – Exploring the factors that contribute to positive outcomes. *International Journal of Adolescence and Youth.* doi:10.1080/02673843.2013.804424.

Deslauriers, J.-M. (2011). Becoming a young father: A decision or an 'accident'? *International Journal of Adolescence and Youth, 16*(3), 289–308.

Dorling, D. (2015). *Social, political, economic and health inequality and our grandchildren's future.* BSA Medical Sociology Group conference, University of York.

Du Bois-Reymond, M. (1998). 'I don't want to commit myself yet': Young people's life concepts. *Journal of Youth Studies, 1*(1), 63–79.

Edin, K., & Kefalas, M. (2005). *Promises I can keep. Why poor women put motherhood before marriage.* Berkeley: University of California Press.

Furlong, A., & Cartmel, F. (2007). *Young people and social change: New perspectives.* Milton Keynes: Open University Press.

Heelas, P., Lash, S., & Morris, P. (Eds.). (1996). *Detraditionalization.* Oxford: Blackwell Publishers.

Hosie, A. C. S. (2007). 'I hated everything about school': An examination of the relationship between dislike of school, teenage pregnancy and educational disengagement. *Social Policy and Society, 6*(3), 333–347.

Kelly, D. (2000). *Pregnant with meaning: Teen mothers and the politics of inclusive schooling.* New York: Peter Lang Publishing.

Kirkman, M., Harrison, M., Hillier, L., & Pyett, P. (2001). 'I know I'm doing a good job': Canonical and autobiographical narratives of teenage mothers. *Culture, Health and Sexuality, 3*(3), 279–294.

Luttrell, W. (2003). *Pregnant bodies, fertile minds: Gender, race and the schooling of pregnant teens.* New York: Routledge.

MacDonald, R. (2006). Social exclusion, youth transitions and criminal careers: Five critical reflections on 'risk'. *Australian and New Zealand Journal of Criminology, 39*(3), 371–383.

MacDonald, R., & Shildrick, T. (2007). Street corner society. *Leisure Studies, 26*(3), 339–55.

MacDonald, R., Shildrick, T., Webster, C., & Simpson, D. (2005). Growing up in poor neighbourhoods: The significance of class and place in the extended transitions of 'socially excluded' young adults. *Sociology, 39*(5), 873–891.

Maruna, S. (2001). *Making good: How ex-convicts reform and rebuild their lives.* Washington, DC: American Psychological Association.

Mason, R., & Wintour, P. (2013). David Cameron admits ministers must 'do far more' to increase social mobility. *The Guardian* newspaper. Retrieved September 30, 2015, from http://www.theguardian.com/society/2013/nov/14/david-cameron-social-mobility-major

McDermott, E., & Graham, H. (2005). Resilient young mothering: Social inequalities, late modernity and the 'problem' of 'teenage' motherhood. *Journal of Youth Studies, 8*(1), 59–79.

McNight, A. (2015). *Downward mobility, opportunity hoarding and the 'glass floor'.* London: Social Mobility and Child Poverty Commission.

McRobbie, A. (2009). *The aftermath of feminism: Gender, culture and social change.* London: Sage.

Mitchell, W., & Green, E. (2002). 'I don't know what I'd do without our Mam' motherhood, identity and support networks. *The Sociological Review, 50,* 1–22.

Nilsen, A., & Brannen, J. (2002). Theorising the individual-structure dynamic. In J. Brannen, S. Lewis, A. Nilsen, & J. Smithson (Eds.), *Young Europeans, work and family: Futures in transition.* London: Routledge.

Phoenix, A. (1991). *Young mothers.* Cambridge: Polity Press.

Rolfe, A. (2008). 'You've got to grow up when you've got a kid': Marginalized young women's accounts of motherhood. *Journal of Community and Applied Social Psychology, 18,* 299–314.

Romagnoli, A., & Wall, G. (2012). 'I know I'm a good mom': Young, low income mothers' experiences with risk perception, intensive parenting ideology and parenting education programmes. *Health, Risk and Society, 14*(3), 273–289.

Shildrick, T., MacDonald, R., Webster, C., & Garthwaite, K. (2012). *Poverty and insecurity: Life in low-pay, no-pay Britain*. Bristol: Policy Press.

SmithBattle, L. (2007). 'I wanna have a good future': Teen mothers' rise in educational aspirations, competing demands and limited school support. *Youth and Society, 38*(3), 348–371.

Social Exclusion Unit (SEU). (1999). *Teenage pregnancy*. London: Stationery Office.

Thomson, R. (2000). Dream on: The logic of sexual practice. *Journal of Youth Studies, 3*(4), 407–427.

Thomson, R., Bell, R., Holland, J., Henderson, S., McGrellis, S., & Sharpe, S. (2002). Critical moments: Choice, chance and opportunity in young people's narratives of transition. *Sociology, 36*(2), 335–354.

Thomson, R., Henderson, S., & Holland, J. (2003). Making the most of what you've got? Resources, values and inequalities in young people's transitions to adulthood. *Educational Review, 55*(1), 33–46.

Thomson, R., & Holland, J. (2002). Imagining adulthood: Resources, plans and contradictions. *Gender and Education, 14*(4), 337–350.

Thomson, R., Holland, J., McGrellis, S., Bell, R., Henderson, S., & Sharpe, S. (2004). Inventing adulthoods: A biographical approach to understanding youth citizenship. *The Sociological Review, 52*(2), 218–239.

Thomson, R., Kehily, M. J., Hadfield, L., & Sharpe, S. (2011). *Making modern mothers*. Bristol: Policy Press.

Tuffin, K., Rouch, G., & Frewin, K. (2010). Constructing adolescent fatherhood: Responsibilities and intergenerational repair. *Culture, Health and Sexuality, 12*(5), 485–498.

Vincent, K., & Thomson, P. (2010). 'Slappers like you don't belong in this school': The educational inclusion/exclusion of pregnant schoolgirls. *International Journal of Inclusive Education, 14*(4), 371–385.

Walkerdine, V., Lucey, H., & Melody, J. (2001). *Growing-up girl: Psycho-social explorations of gender and class*. London: Palgrave.

Yardley, E. (2009). Teenage mothers' experiences of formal support services. *Journal of Social Policy, 38*(2), 241–257.

9

'My Mum is a Young Mum and She's Done Fine': Conclusions

The purposes of The Generations Study were to explore the views and experiences of teenage parenting in families where more than one generation had become parents as teenagers, and to discuss how decisions were made about whether or not to become a mother or father. Through formal interviews and focus groups, casual conversations that happen before and after the recorder is running, and observations taking place while playing with toddlers at drop-in sessions and chatting to their mums, stories have emerged of what it is like to be a teenage parent, what it was like 20 or 50 years ago, and how young parents and those around them feel about how society views them. I began the book by reviewing how some aspects of motherhood have been problematised for well over a century; I end in this concluding chapter by discussing constructions of parenthood and motherhood in social, cultural and policy contexts, and exploring the interactions between the individual biographies of the participants in the study, and the familial and social settings and cultures in which they live. I introduce the analytical concept of 'rewriting the life script', an active process by which young people make sense of themselves and their lives as parents.

© The Editor(s) (if applicable) and The Author(s) 2016   **211**
S. Brown, *Teenage Pregnancy, Parenting and Intergenerational Relations*,
DOI 10.1057/978-1-137-49539-6_9

This chapter will also revisit the international context discussed in Chapter 2, in particular the continuing focus on teenage parenting as a major social problem despite the ongoing decline in the numbers of teenagers having children in most Western-developed nations. I begin by outlining the key themes emerging from the study.

Key Themes

One of the issues that inspired and informed this study is the relationship between generations with the shared experience of becoming a teenage parent, particularly the role of intergenerational transmission; is it something that, as Lydia suggested right at the beginning, runs in families? Murphy (2013) found that intergenerational fertility patterns do occur, with a correlation between the fertility patterns of parents and their children in 28 countries, including the UK, the USA and Canada. In this study, the families that lived close to each other geographically engage in what Brannen calls a 'solidaristic' (2006, p. 140) pattern of intergenerational relations, with parents and grandparents supporting their teenagers in a number of ways: providing accommodation for the teenage mother and her baby until she can find her own home, giving financial support, and helping with childcare. Although the arrival of a baby might fracture some relationships (for example, between the young parents) it also presents an opportunity to mend others (between estranged fathers and daughters). To set the scene for the rest of the discussion, I summarise my findings around the themes that emerged from the study relating to all the generations:

- Unplanned pregnancies
- Family shock and upset, followed by acceptance
- Supportive families (mostly), geographically close
- Interruptions in college or working life
- Becoming a family.

Unplanned Pregnancies

Almost all the pregnancies, across all the generations, were unplanned. A small minority of the current generation of teenagers had actively decided to try to get pregnant, and these tended to be the older ones (Becky aged 18, and Ella aged 19), who were both in stable relationships and planned to get married. None of the others had been intending to get pregnant, although a few said that they had 'always' wanted a baby, so were happy to find that they were expecting. Mostly, the pregnancy was accidental, a shock, and caused the young women to feel upset and frightened about the reaction they would get, from parents, other family members, their wider social circle, and even strangers.

Family (and Other) Reactions

As feared by the young women, their families' first reactions to the announcement of a pregnancy was shock, upset, or even anger. This had been the same for the older generations, although the difference was that none of the younger generation had been asked to move out of the family home by the parents, unlike some of the generation that are now grandparents. However, following on quickly from the upset came acceptance and a willingness to welcome a new baby into the family, if not during the pregnancy then at least once the baby arrived. Most of the older generation looked forward to becoming grandparents, and enjoyed the role, although a few had been reluctant grandparents and took time to accept the baby.

Supportive Families, Geographically Close

Most young parents were part of a relatively large family network that included grandparents, siblings, aunts and uncles, and cousins; for some, many members of the network lived within walking distance, and if not, one or two short bus rides away. Where there had been difficulties within the family home during a pregnancy, for example Paula being asked to leave home by her father, these were often resolved later and family relationships resumed. The current grandparents often wanted their daughters to stay at home, sometimes as a reaction to knowing what it had been like to be asked to leave by their parents, but in other cases repeating their own experience; Sheila had lived with her mother, Eileen, until her son was nearly two, and expected Debbie to carry on living at home once her baby was born.

Interruptions in Education or Work

Far from being a 'negative end point' (Hosie 2007, p. 334) in a teenager's life trajectory, pregnancy and parenthood were incorporated into a life course that for most women would have included children at some point, just perhaps not during their teens (although probably not much later). For those in education, parenthood meant an interruption and a pause; they planned to take, or had taken, a break and would resume their courses when they were ready. For some, this could be quite soon; Debbie planned to go back to college after a break of a few months. Others wanted to wait until their children were at least a year old and they would feel happy leaving them in a nursery. This is one area where there is a clear difference between the older and younger generations. The older generations had either not been at school, or had left as a result of the pregnancy and did not resume education. Most then started working when their children were older. The reason for this difference probably lies in the availability of work for the older generations, particularly the more widespread availability of a range of often part-time care roles that did not demand high qualifications, meaning that work could be fitted around motherhood.

Becoming a Family

Young people actively worked on being a family, whether they took a conventional route with a nuclear family/household overlap, lived as a single adult with their child, or lived in three-generation households. Those in the latter situation looked forward to creating their own household with their partner and baby, and many wished to get married. The proportion of couples marrying has been declining for many years in the UK and the USA. However, this does not necessarily mean that marriage is seen as unimportant; the women in Edin and Kefalas' study (2005) held marriage in such high regard, they argued, that they did not want to commit themselves to it until they were sure their marriage would last. Marriage in this sense confirms stability, but it is also a luxury. The young couples in my study saw marriage as something to wish for and aspire to; they wanted to get married, partly to demonstrate to the outside world that they were stable, but it was expensive so they would wait. Some young people, although not conforming to norms of nuclear families, defined what they did as family in a way that worked for them, such as Katy, who although not living with her son's father, said they were still a family because they undertook family practices, focussed on bringing up their son.

Constructions of Parenthood

Chapter 2 showed how certain types of mothers (unmarried, lone or young) have been regarded as problematic and in need of regulation and control at various times through the last century and beyond. The fathers involved with those women have often been regarded as feckless and irresponsible, and in need of coercion to oblige them to face up to their responsibilities, for example, via the metaphorical shotgun leading to a wedding, or by state agencies enforcing child support payments. As well as a policy focus on motherhood, research has largely focussed on mothers, and a great deal more has been written about them than about fathers. Indeed, more women than men took part in my study, so much more can be said about how women think and feel about motherhood than can be said about men and fatherhood. The next section of this chapter considers how parenthood is constructed in social, cultural and policy contexts. Here, I introduce the concept of 'rewriting the life script', an active process which young people undertake to make sense of themselves and their lives as parents.

Social and Cultural Contexts of Parenthood

Parenthood can be viewed in a number of ways; in a social context, it operates in terms of how an individual takes on the role as a mother or father, how it affects their lives and how they construct their new identity as a parent, if indeed they do. One of the reasons for there being fewer male than female participants in this study was due to young women taking part who were raising their babies by themselves, because their former partners had ended the relationship, either during the pregnancy or shortly after the baby was born. In denying that a baby is his, or by ending a relationship, a young man can opt out of parenthood and refuse to take on the identity of being a father in a way that young women cannot. Even where a woman gives her baby up for adoption, she often retains an identity as a mother herself, even if other people might not know about it, as some of the films and literature discussed in Chapter 2 demonstrate.

In talking about the cultural context of parenthood, I use culture to mean everyday social practice (Thomson et al. 2011), in this case relating to families, and in particular, maternal cultures created by successive generations of women, who shape themselves as like or unlike earlier generations. Despite critiques from some feminist writers of the roles of families as social institutions, family remains important to many people as part of their everyday activities. Family practices (Morgan 2013), in terms of the everyday doing of family, create a cultural context within which mothers (and fathers) act, and in this setting, a cultural context where children are valued. Edin and Kefalas (2005) suggest that the working-class women in their study, based in Philadelphia, value children more than middle-class women, largely because their children are at the 'centre of their meaning making activity' (2005, p. 206), rather than education or career. In their study of families living in poverty in Northern Ireland, Daly and Kelly (2015) found that parents have an identity that is invested in their children, and even where they have had bad experiences of family, make great efforts to create ideal family relationships, largely through their children. Young mothers, like older ones, are proud of their children and try to put them first (Owen et al. 2010; Phoenix 1991), in many cases going without themselves in order to ensure their children's needs are met (Daly and

Kelly 2015). These studies demonstrate remarkable consistencies across place (USA and UK) and time in terms of the continued importance of family, and how much children mean to parents.

Rewriting the Life Script

For the young women in my study, motherhood was a critical moment (Thomson et al. 2002) at which they made the transition from teenager, to mother, and adult. This was a point at which they rewrote their life script as part of taking on an identity of 'mother'. As Kehily points out, motherhood is 'a moment of profound identity change' (2009, p. 5) for all women regardless of age, and in many ways teenagers are no different to older mothers. They face many of the same challenges, as well as specific ones relating to their age, which I will come to shortly. But for most, they are 'just a mum or dad' (Alexander et al. 2010, p. 135), and they either do not see themselves as part of the problematic group of 'young parents' (like the older teens in Bridgetown), or they actively reject the stigmatising process whereby 'teenage parent' equals 'bad parent'.

Rewriting the life script takes two routes. Firstly there are those who, like Naomi, had a life script of education (sixth form, plans for university) and career (ambition to become a teacher) which was knocked off course by an unexpected pregnancy. Not feeling that abortion or adoption were acceptable options for her, she and her partner Jamie had their baby, found a house, and settled down with plans to marry. Naomi's educational ambitions shifted to hairdressing, a course she could cope with at college, and she threw her energies into being a mother, saying she 'wouldn't change it for the world', and a homemaker, seeing her role as running the household, making sure everyone was happy, and supporting Jamie in his ambition to get a university place and become a teacher. Naomi's rewritten life script shifts her away from her original ambitions and replaces them with a new script with which she is happy.

As has been noted previously, Naomi was unusual amongst the young mothers in that she had plans for university and a career. The second route to rewriting the life script was much more common, and took the form of embracing motherhood as a way of gaining a role and a positive identity. For some, such as Megan, who did poorly at school, and who, at 15 years old, had no clear ideas or plans about what she might do in life, motherhood was an identity and role she could embrace and where she could feel pride, both in her abilities to manage her own household, and in her children. From being uncertain and describing herself as lacking in confidence, she gains an identity and can talk about herself as a mother, and as someone who is doing well, feels settled, and is approaching her seventh anniversary with her partner, which she sees as a sign of success and achievement.

We often ask children and young teenagers 'what do you want to do when you grow up?' with the unspoken assumption that the question relates to future employment; in other words, suggesting that knowing what to 'do', and then doing it in terms of getting the desired job, marks the transition to adulthood. Young people in the study often talked about not knowing what they wanted to do before they had children, and here parenthood clearly acts as a point of transition, a point at which they can write themselves a new life script where they do know what they want to do, because now they have a reason. For those who had been unsure about what they wanted to do, rewriting their life script meant being able to say that now they were a mother, they had a reason to complete a college course, get qualifications that they previously would not have aimed for, and ultimately to find a good job that would mean they could support their family and have a stable and secure home. Katy's rewritten life script incorporates this turning point and she explicitly states that becoming a mother gave her the reason and the opportunity to think about what she wanted to do, and to write a life script that includes completing NVQs as part of an apprenticeship, and having obtained qualifications, carrying on to become a youth worker. Other aspects incorporated into a rewritten life script include being a more sensible person now, or being responsible. Haley, for example, describes herself as taking fewer risks and sees having a baby to come home to as a sign that she has changed her life for the better.

One of the striking aspects of the way many of the young women talk about their lives is how many of them embrace a traditional approach to motherhood, gendered roles and family, Naomi being a prime example. Thomson and Holland found that the majority of young people in their study followed a normative model of career, marriage and family by the age of 35, and suggest that they are 'constrained by a resilient model of adulthood anchored in heteronormative notions of "settling down"' (2002, p. 348). They argue that youth transitions are fluid, but that they remain structured by class and gender as well as by race and locality, and this seems to be the case for a majority of participants in this study, of all generations.

Young men also rewrite their life scripts as fathers. Some, like Steve, incorporate an element of the redemption script (Maruna 2001) in turning away from a previous self and taking on a new identity as a responsible father who will put his child first. The young fathers also talked in terms of a traditional breadwinner model whereby they are working or hope to work, and wish to support their families. Some couples, like Steve and Ella, plan that he will find a job and she will stay at home with their son until he is of school age. Carl wished to earn enough to make sure he could provide for his family, while leaving the running of the household to Becky. As we saw in Chapter 8, for Carl and Dave, fatherhood meant 'doing dad things' that can be thought of as having a traditional aspect, such as gardening and making sure their children did their homework, as well as taking on caring roles for their partner (making her cups of tea and looking after her when she was breast-feeding, as Dave did for Jenny). Like the young men in MacDonald and Marsh's Teesside study, young fathers 'express sentiments and aspire to lead lives quite at odds with the mean portraits of "absent fathers" offered in the underclass literature' (2005, p. 141). The rewritten life script for young fathers, then, is one where they are responsible, sensible, and caring, and where, as for the mothers, their children become their priority.

Countering a Stigmatising Identity

There may, of course, be an element of performance in the way that the young parents present themselves as happy and as embracing their rewritten life script; they may feel regret for what they have left behind, in terms of a carefree adolescence without responsibilities, but feel the need to act out an identity within an interview or focus group. However, they did not present their lives as problem free; many of them talked about hardship, whether financial or in terms of the hard work of being a parent. Some mentioned loneliness and almost all of them talked about being judged and stigmatised as young parents, and how bad that made them feel. Young people are well aware of the overwhelmingly negative discourses of teenage pregnancy and parenting, and are 'highly attuned to what people thought of them' (Wenham 2015, p. 9), expecting disapproval, derogatory comments and 'mucky looks' whenever they go out. Arai argues 'that there are few population subgroups who appear to embody so many social and moral evils' (2009, p. 48) in the way they are depicted and described, with teenage mothers often portrayed as an underclass apart from mainstream society (Alexander et al. 2010). As Luttrell (2003) shows, young mothers cannot fashion a sense of self that ignores the dominant discourses about teenage parenting, but they can apply individual agency in the way they represent themselves. The young women in this study acknowledge the dominant discourses, that teenage motherhood is bad, that it means people will be on benefits for life, and then define themselves as opposite to that; they are good mothers, they do not intend to be on benefits for ever, they have aspirations. In their rewritten life scripts, they present themselves as clearly not the stigmatised version of 'teenage mother'. Like the young women in Shea et al.'s (2015) study, by exercising agency and thus imbuing their lives with purpose and meaning, the young parents here distance themselves from the negative stereotypes. Stigma and judgement play such a big role in the lives of young parents that they have to write themselves a life script focussing on a positive sense of identity in order to counter that. No-one could live within that stigmatised identity and retain any sense of self-worth or value.

The cultural representation of teenage parenting is one where teenage mothers are positioned as irresponsible, bad parents, and a drain on society, and young fathers are portrayed as feckless at best, and at worst a danger to their children. The young parents in this study work hard to present themselves as good mothers and fathers in order to place themselves as 'other' to the stereotypes of teenage parents. They acknowledge the label, and as we saw earlier, by using a 'bad people exist but I'm not one of them' discourse (Kingfisher 1996, p. 56) distance themselves from it. They go to great lengths to provide a visual image of good parenting by thinking about how they dress, how their baby is dressed, and how they appear to the outside world, demonstrating respectability by showing how accomplished they are at caring (Skeggs 1997) as a necessary part of proving that they are good, and not as Naomi said, 'bad parents, bad *people*'. Wenham (2015) describes how the young mothers in her study felt under pressure to prove themselves as differing from the stereotype, and for some of the young parents in my study this pressure meant ensuring that no-one could look down on them for their or their baby's appearance.

Social and Cultural Capital

As members of a stigmatised group, whose pregnancies are said to result from irresponsible or ignorant behaviour, who are dependent on the state, and who have only 'shattered lives and blighted futures' (SEU 1999) to look forward to, teenage parents have almost no economic, social or cultural capital as far as wider society is concerned. In societies governed by neoliberal ideals of individualism and the primacy of economic goals, teenage parents who appear to have chosen a path other than one of maximising their earnings potential are going against the neoliberal discourse of success coming through education and labour market participation (McRobbie 2009). However, this ignores two points. Firstly, as has been shown, for the groups most likely to become teenage parents (in any of countries within Chandola et al.'s (2002) 'anglophone' grouping, not just the USA and the UK), having a child early has little to no effect on their later earnings potential. Middle-class women, who are more likely to continue their education and to invest in a career, have very different opportunity costs of lost future earnings if they have children early and interrupt their career, compared to working-class women who have a similar earnings trajectory regardless of when they have children (Hotz et al. 1996; Geronimus 1997; Edin and Kefalas 2005). Where career and economic goals have primacy, having a baby is talked about in terms of interrupting a career. Where family is important, work is something that is fitted around children.

Secondly, they are living in a context where family and children have primacy over individualist economic goals; in this setting, or in Bourdieu's language, field, they have considerable social capital, because they are doing something that is valued when they produce the next generation. Walkerdine et al. highlight the importance of the 'situated and specifically local character of how people live' (2001, p. 15) and here, the local cultural contexts within which most young parents live is one where children are highly valued. Motherhood is a valued and respectable role, and grandparenthood is something to be anticipated with pleasure, and enjoyed. In this sense, from being a teenager who is disengaged from school or not doing very well, who is unlikely to get a good job or cannot find any work, all factors which contribute to having little social or economic capital, parenthood enhances their capitals. As Thomson (2000) argues, young women gain capital from the experience and authority of motherhood, but this has little value outside their social setting. Therefore, they need to enhance their capitals in other ways as well, and this is via education, for which parenthood has provided an incentive.

Being educated is part of having cultural capital, as well as enhancing potential for improving economic capital. We have seen the importance of education for the young people involved in this study, including those who have previously been disaffected. A culture of self-improvement informs a view of parenthood as a turning point that many of the young parents subscribed to, particularly in terms of getting an education for the baby's sake. Both cultural and economic capital are also enhanced where work is an essential aspect of a self-improvement narrative, as it leads to economic independence and a move away from dependency on benefits.

The Policy Context

Chapter 2 showed that UK governments have had an interest in families for over a century, and have created a range of social policies over time that have attempted to manage families and family life in a way that meets particular policy objectives of that government. For example, in the early years of the twentieth century, the concern with public health and the future health of the nation resulted in state support for mothers (Thane and Evans 2012). More recently, the New Labour governments of 1997–2010 made family policy central to their views on citizenship and social inclusion, largely through emphasising the need to participate in the workplace in order to be a fully competent citizen. Defining citizenship as based around these two axes, of inclusion/exclusion and work/worklessness (Tyler 2013, p. 161), means in effect that being employed means being part of mainstream society, and everything else equals dependency. As Daly and Kelly (2015) point out, ideas about what constitutes a good family are prominent in social policy, with the emphasis being very much on a good family being one that is self-sufficient, where people 'rely more on themselves and their families, and less on the state' (2015, p. 5). They criticise the individualistic approach to poverty, whereby it is only people's lack of agency that keeps them poor, as this ignores the structural constraints that limit the choices people can make.

As we saw with the TPS, teenage pregnancy was very clearly linked to social exclusion, but this is in a context where parenthood is not seen as a valued role, and not acknowledged as being a component of social inclusion. Edwards et al. (2010) suggest that policies that focus on employment being the only way to make a contribution to society assume the opposite of what teenage parenting actually means to some young people. Such policies fail to see that for those young people for whom 'being a mother or father can make good sense' (Edwards et al. 2010, p. 199), parenthood can act as an incentive, motivating them to improve their lives. The young people in this study have demonstrated that this is the case many times.

Under the Coalition government of 2010–2015 the focus on the family remained, but shifted to concentrate more closely on the 'problem families' who supposedly make up 'Broken Britain'. Although teenage parents are mentioned in some of the Troubled Families documentation, there are no specific targets relating to teenage parents within the Troubled Families programme (DCLG 2012a, 2012b). The focus on troubled families has retained a central place in social policy for the current Conservative government, with the extension of the Troubled Families programme being announced in the Queen's Speech in May 2015.

International Perspectives

Chapter 2 provided a comparative perspective on teenage pregnancy as an issue, and focussed particularly on the five anglophone nations that the UNICEF report in 2001 highlighted as having the highest rates amongst the developed nations of the world. The UK has had high teenage pregnancy rates compared to other Western European countries, but they are similar to those of Australia, New Zealand and Canada, with the USA having the highest rates of the five. Although the rates remain high compared to many Western European and Asian nations, they have been declining in all five countries for a number of years.

The approach to teenage pregnancy, in policy terms, is similar across the anglophone countries in that it is regarded as a problem to be solved. Chapter 2 outlined the focus placed on teenage pregnancy in the UK, particularly during the New Labour years, as an issue of social exclusion. Currently, the reduction of teenage pregnancy rates is one of the Department of Health's *Public Health Outcomes Framework* targets linked to reducing poverty; as health is a devolved issue in the UK, this applies to England only. In Wales, reducing teenage pregnancy has been part of the sexual health strategy, and in Scotland it is also part of the strategy for improving sexual health. In New Zealand, reducing unplanned pregnancies, including teenage pregnancies, is part of the Sexual and Reproductive Health Strategy (Ministry of Health 2001). At national level in the USA, reducing teenage pregnancy is one of six top priorities for public health, and regarded as one of the 'winnable battles' in public health terms (CDC 2015). President Obama initiated the Teen Pregnancy Prevention Initiative (TPPI) in 2010 with $110 million of competitive contracts and grants to public and private bodies, for 'medically accurate and age-appropriate programs that reduce teen pregnancy and associated risk behaviours' (personal communication). However, the desire to reduce teenage pregnancy rates is not matched by a national strategy in the way it was in the UK, not least due to the federal system of government in the USA, where it is up to individual states to decide how to implement policies. The Department of Health and Human Services Office of Adolescent Health runs an evidence-based teen pregnancy prevention program, but again, this is not a nationwide strategy, but a collection of initiatives that service providers can apply for in order to run programmes at state or community level; however, it is a competitive process and not all who apply will receive funding. On top of the national schemes, some states have their own teen pregnancy prevention funding.

Although the relatively high teenage pregnancy rates are issues of concern for the governments of Australia and Canada, there are currently no overarching national policy initiatives or strategies for reducing rates. Like the USA, they have federal government systems, and health policies are made at provincial and state levels; where there are policies relating to teenage pregnancy, for example in Ontario in Canada and Victoria in Australia, they fall within the remit of sexual health service provision. Between 2005 and 2007 the Public Health Agency of Canada had the reduction of teen pregnancy in Canada as one of its four priorities, and as part of this ran *On the Move* initiative which aimed to enable communities to take action to reduce teen pregnancy rates. Again, the actual programmes were decided by individual provinces.

What links the USA and the UK most closely is a government approach based on tackling welfare dependency, predicated on ideas about the existence of an underclass whose members choose to give birth at an early age, not to marry, and to opt for a life on benefits rather than work. However, a great deal of what has been said about the existence of an underclass has been challenged. Welshman provides a very thorough and detailed discussion of the development of theories about the underclass in the USA and the UK, ultimately describing it as 'a convenient symbol and metaphor for fears and anxieties whose empirical reality remains unproven' (Welshman 2006, p. 210). Tyler argues that the creation of 'national abjects' who become 'symbolic and material scapegoats' (2013, p. 9) is a way for neoliberal governments to create consent for the increasing restriction of any form of state support for those who are thus labelled. Teenage parents are amongst those who are scapegoated as both cause and effect of a failed welfare state in the UK and the USA, with

Formby et al. (2010) arguing that the media sustain inaccurate portrayals of young parents, which feeds into Tyler's process of abjection.

Policy approaches, then, almost always start from a negative perspective and rarely consider any positive aspects of teenage parenthood. Given the growth in qualitative research which takes a different perspective, there is now a strong body of work which challenges this. As well as the growing body of UK based research (for example, Rolfe 2008; Arai 2009; Duncan et al. 2010; Middleton 2011), American writers such as Lee SmithBattle, Frank Furstenberg and Arline Geronimus are amongst those making a case that for many young women, parenthood is a positive experience, as do Brand et al. (2015) in Australia; evidence from Canada (Deslauriers 2011) and New Zealand (Tuffin et al. 2010) finds that this holds true for young fathers. Across these five anglophone countries with the highest rates and problematising policy approaches, there is qualitative evidence from young people that is at odds with what policymakers would have us believe.

The social exclusion approach, whereby reducing rates of teenage pregnancy will reduce social exclusion, and fewer children will grow up in poor homes if there are fewer teenage parents, has become the dominant policy discourse across the anglophone countries, However, while preventing teenage pregnancy is one of the tools for reducing poverty, as in England's *Public Health Outcomes Framework*, as Furstenberg asks, 'the reverse is rarely given consideration: how do we prevent poverty and social disadvantage as a way of reducing early childbearing?' (2007, p. 52).

Where Next? The Future, Policy and Practice

Wilson and Huntington (2006) point out the paradox of teenage pregnancy being a major concern in many developed countries at a point when rates have been falling for many years. As Table 2.1 showed in Chapter 2, the five anglophone countries I have focussed on all experienced significant falls between 1999 and 2013, and similar declines can be seen in most European countries. Their argument is that as 'middle-class aspirations for well-paid professional jobs have come to set the parameters for social inclusion' (2006, p. 69), life trajectories that deviate from this path are seen as socially excluded; the solution, then, is for the excluded to become more like the included. As Geronimus argues, a rather naive view of how to solve the problem of high teenage pregnancy rates in the USA seems to suggest that 'if African Americans adopt the nuclear family and delayed fertility norms of European Americans, this alone would induce social, economic and political equality' (2003, p. 882). A similar line of thought seems to inform UK social policy: if only working-class girls could be more like middle-class ones, stay on at school and get good jobs, teenage pregnancy and all sorts of other social ills would disappear. However, rather than addressing Furstenberg's argument that we should be focussing on addressing poverty and disadvantage and its causal relationship with teenage pregnancy, it is likely that the economic approach taken by the anglophone governments will continue to place economic success above caring and parenting as valuable social roles. In addition, the ideologically driven austerity approach to the welfare state in the UK in particular means that state support for people unable to find work, or able only to find low-paid, unstable work, will become harder to access, and minimal in the support it provides if it can be accessed. Indeed, the impact assessment carried out by the Department for Work and Pensions into the welfare reforms proposed in the 2015 Budget and the Welfare Reform and Work Bill 2015 suggested that single mothers will be the group most affected by these changes.

One of the effects of the benefit cap, introduced in an earlier budget and intended to ensure that no family can receive more in state support than the average family in work, has been to make parts of the country unaffordable for unemployed people, as benefits no longer cover the costs of renting, particularly in parts of London. The impact of the lower cap introduced by the 2015 budget will extend this area to large parts of the south of England, as well as some northern cities. This means that people affected will have to move to a cheaper part of the country. For many families, this means not only significant disruption to children's schooling and contact with wider family, but it will also have major implications in terms of how families can manage their lives. As the discussion earlier has shown, young parents do not, for the most part, exist in isolation; they are part of supportive families, and that practical family support enables them to continue their education, and once they find a job, enables them to work. The types of jobs that the young parents can find tend to be low-paid and insecure, which means that childcare is often unaffordable or impractical, childminders and nurseries generally requiring several weeks' notice to book the sessions required. Therefore, family support, mostly in the form of childcare by grandparents, is an essential component in enabling young parents to train and work. If the effect of the benefit cap is to require them to move away from their family networks, then they are less likely to be able to work. Despite the Secretary of State for Work and Pensions, Iain Duncan Smith, saying that the benefit cap incentivises 'behaviour change', in other words getting a job, there is little evidence that it does. Life is likely to get harder for young parents in the next few years as the austerity agenda makes policies more punitive at a time when young people are facing challenges; as Stapleton (2010) suggests, there is a need for support rather than policing at that point in their lives.

Is There such a Thing as Intergenerational Transmission?

Alexander et al. suggest that teenage parenthood is 'emblematic of an "underclass" which is outside of mainstream British society, and which is defined through pathologised moral and cultural values, "lifestyles and behaviour", seemingly transmitted across generations' (2010, p. 136). From the perspective of those who support an underclass or cycle of deprivation thesis, there is a view that it is, as Arai so vividly writes, 'a kind of blight with a viral-like nature … capable of spreading itself through a youthful population and able to withstand efforts to defeat it' (2009, p. 48).

However, there is some evidence that children's fertility patterns are correlated with those of their parents (Murphy 2013); in other words, children are often like their parents, which is unsurprising. There is also some evidence, much of it American, that daughters of teenage mothers are more likely to become young mothers, as are the sisters of teenage mothers. The question is, why might children follow in the footsteps of their parents, particularly in terms of when they have their own families, and particularly where, like the families who have told their stories in this book, there was such a strong desire on the part of the parents for their children not to follow in their footsteps? Underclass theorists would have us believe that, as Arai and Alexander et al. wrote, it is some kind of virus transmitted from parent to child that causes them to become a teenage mother. However, I would argue that the connection is not about getting pregnant, but about the decision-making process once a teenager is pregnant. Mothers were insistent that they had given their daughters strong guidance about not getting pregnant at a young age, and about using contraception, and we have seen how worried the young women were about telling their parents about their pregnancy. Clearly, they did not expect their announcement to be welcome news and had not felt any encouragement to become pregnant. However, once a young woman is pregnant, she looks to those around her; where her mother, possibly her grandmother, and maybe also her sisters have been teenage mothers, there is evidence that teenage mothers manage, so she probably will manage as well. Where family is valued, role models are other family members. Where experience shows that teenage parenting is not the disaster that politicians would have us believe, young people are more likely to take heed of the experience that they know. Haley knows 'it isn't the end of the world' because her mother was a mother at 14, and both her older sisters had had children by the time they were 17. The other factor is that for a lot of the young women, they do not consider an abortion to be an option. They are not opposed to it entirely, just for themselves. For Zara, having an abortion when other family members were unable to have children would be letting the family down. The teenagers, for the most part, are not acting in isolation—they are part of a family, and their decisions are made in that family and social context.

Conclusions

The research discussed in this book has shown the contradictions inherent in a policy approach that sees teenage pregnancy and parenthood as universally negative, and a destructive experience which causes problems, whilst lived experience provides somewhat different evidence. This accords with Graham and McDermott (2006) and their suggestion that the different results of quantitative and qualitative work are on the one hand accepted (quantitative studies) and on the other disregarded (qualitative studies), not least because they fit to a greater or lesser extent with the desired policy approach. Furstenberg argued in 2003 that 'political and public perceptions of teenage childbearing have not kept pace with either the dramatic declines in teenage childbearing rates or the research on the consequences of teenage births' (2003, p. 34) and much of the evidence from the media, politicians and public opinion which has appeared throughout this book would seem to indicate that this is as true for the UK in 2015 as it was for the USA in 2003.

Many studies have compared different attitudes towards sex and sexual openness between countries such as the Netherlands, France, Australia, and the USA (Weaver et al. 2005), Canada, Sweden, France, Great Britain and the USA (Singh et al. 2001), Nordic and Southern European countries (Træen et al. 2011), and across Europe (Imamura et al. 2007). There appears to be a consensus that societies with more open and liberal attitudes towards sex alongside comprehensive and pragmatic sex education and access to non-judgemental sexual health services have much lower teenage pregnancy rates, as well as better sexual health, than countries (mainly the USA) that focus on abstinence education. Lottes (2002) suggested that the non-judgemental attitudes of the Netherlands and the Nordic countries to teenage sexuality means that teenagers in those countries are more empowered than those in the USA and therefore are better able to negotiate the use of contraception. Whilst access to contraception and comprehensive sex education have an impact on lowering rates (Singh et al. 2001; Blackman 2013), the pace of economic change and the degree of income inequality seem to have determined the speed and magnitude of the reductions across a wide range of countries (Sedgh et al. 2015), with socio-economic and demographic factors being critical (Girma and Paton 2015). As teenage pregnancy rates are highest in countries with the greatest degrees of income inequality (UK and USA), and the UK is on track to become the most unequal country in the world by 2020 (Dorling 2015), it remains to be seen whether the growing disparities in the UK will have an impact on rates, or whether the downward trend will continue.

The localities featured in this book have been affected by global processes that have led to decline and deindustrialisation, and this impacts on continuities and discontinuities in the lives of individuals. We have seen how important the continuity of family and family practices are to the people who have told their stories. Industrial decline means that aspects of life that were once certain are no longer supported; pregnancy, children, a settled home, and a family to be provided for were continuities that past generations, such as the older generations of the Baker and Jones families, could rely on. It is something that the younger generations— Carl and Becky, Steve and Ella—would very much like. Global recession has not meant the end of work, but it has meant the end of stability for huge numbers of people. If one can never be sure of securing stability, waiting to be stable before having a child makes no sense.

Young people are frequently positioned in terms of being unwise or unaware of their best interests, and characterised as making choices that do not fit with desirable social norms, regardless of whether it could be objectively assessed to be a rational choice. In fact in families where there is a history of young motherhood, keeping the baby is for many a rational choice, with proof existing in the family that it is a good choice; for some it becomes a turning point and for others is an interruption but still acts as an incentive to succeed.

We have seen a shift from viewing unwed motherhood as a moral problem to seeing teenage motherhood as a social problem. As such, it is framed in an approach that looks at the cumulative risks of young parenting, and in health terms frames them in a discourse about inequality and disadvantage. Thus teenage motherhood is positioned as a problem to be solved, largely by individualised measures that do little to address any underlying influences. SmithBattle (2012) credits the 'upstream policies' of France, Sweden and Denmark with creating low levels of social disadvantage and consequently low rates of teenage pregnancy. She also highlights the pre-2010 approach in the UK in supporting low income families as one which does address underlying issues of poverty and disadvantage.

Wilson and Huntington (2006) suggest that policy approaches to teenage parenting in the USA, the UK and New Zealand, which focus on social exclusion and welfare dependency, are obscuring the ideological and class-based nature of policies which in effect punish teenage mothers for not conforming to middle-class trajectories of higher education and workforce participation. In the current neoliberal climate, young women are expected to take up educational opportunities, pursue a career and become part of consumer culture (McRobbie 2009), but teenage parenthood acts as a denial of this. Furthermore, when fertility is regarded as something under control, teenage pregnancy is a failure of control which damages the young woman's status as a responsible citizen (Fallon 2010).

This book has tried to tell a story about the lives of young parents across the generations. Like Walkerdine et al. (2001) finding that the position of young women in the new economy is uncomfortable, the position of young parents in the modern economy is difficult and tenuous. Caught in situations often not of their own making, they are blamed for not making better situations but given few tools with which to dig themselves out, despite appearing to want very much the independence, economic stability and a happy family life that, as members of a so-called underclass, they are supposed to be undermining. By rewriting their life scripts, they challenge the stigmatised identity of 'teenage parent' and position themselves as good parents with a strong commitment to their children and to family life. It is not vilification that they deserve, but commendation for doing a good job and support for to ensure they and their children have secure futures.

References

Alexander, C., Duncan, S., & Edwards, R. (2010). 'Just a mum or dad': Experiencing teenage parenting and work-life balance. In S. Duncan, R. Edwards, & C. Alexander (Eds.), *Teenage parenthood: What's the problem?* London: Tuffnell Press.

Arai, L. (2009). *Teenage pregnancy: The making and unmaking of a problem.* Bristol: Policy Press.

Blackman, T. (2013). Exploring explanations for local reductions in teenage pregnancy rates in England: An approach using qualitative comparative analysis. *Social Policy and Society, 12*(1), 61–72.

Brand, G., Morrison, P., & Down, B. (2015). 'You don't know half the story': Deepening the dialogue with young mothers in Australia. *Journal of Research in Nursing.* doi:10.1177/1744987114565223.

Brannen, J. (2006). Cultures of intergenerational transmission in four-generation families. *The Sociological Review, 54*(1), 133–154.

Centres for Disease Control and Prevention (CDC). (2015). *Winnable battles.* Retrieved 30, 2015, from http://www.cdc.gov/winnablebattles/

Chandola, T., Coleman, D. A., & Hiorns, R. W. (2002). Heterogeneous fertility patterns in the English-speaking world. Results from Australia, Canada, New Zealand and the United States. *Population Studies, 56*(2), 181–200.

Daly, M., & Kelly, G. (2015). *Families and poverty. Everyday life on a low income.* Bristol: Policy Press.

Department for Communities and Local Government. (2012a). *Financial framework for the Troubled Families programme's payment-by-results scheme for local authorities.* London: DCLG.

Department for Communities and Local Government. (2012b). *Listening to troubled families: A report by Louise Casey CBE.* London: DCLG.

Deslauriers, J.-M. (2011). Becoming a young father: A decision or an 'accident'? *International Journal of Adolescence and Youth, 16*(3), 289–308.

Dorling, D. (2015). *Social, political, economic and health inequality and our grandchildren's future.* BSA Medical Sociology Group conference, University of York.

Duncan, S., Edwards, R., & Alexander, C. (Eds.). (2010). *Teenage parenthood: What's the problem?* London: Tuffnell Press.

Edin, K., & Kefalas, M. (2005). *Promises I can keep. Why poor women put motherhood before marriage.* Berkeley: University of California Press.

Edwards, R., Duncan, S., & Alexander, C. (2010). Conclusion: Hazard warning. In S. Duncan, R. Edwards, & C. Alexander (Eds.), *Teenage parenthood: What's the problem?* London: Tuffnell Press.

Fallon, D. (2010). Accessing emergency contraception: The role of friends in the adolescent experience. *Sociology of Health and Illness, 32*(5), 677–694.

Formby, E., Hirst, J., & Owen, J. (2010). Pathways to adulthood: Reflections from three generations of young mothers. In S. Duncan, R. Edwards, & C. Alexander (Eds.), *Teenage parenthood: What's the problem?* London: Tuffnell Press.

Furstenberg, F. (2003). Teenage childbearing as a public issue and private concern. *Annual Review of Sociology, 29*, 23–39.

Furstenberg, F. (2007). *Destinies of the disadvantaged. The politics of teenage childbearing.* New York: Russell Sage Foundation.

Geronimus, A. T. (1997). Teenage childbearing and personal responsibility: An alternative view. *Political Science Quarterly, 112*(3), 405–430.

Geronimus, A. T. (2003). Damned if you do: Culture, identity, privilege, and teenage childbearing in the United States. *Social Science and Medicine, 57*, 881–893.

Girma, S., & Paton, D. (2015). Is education the best contraception: The case of teenage pregnancy in England? *Social Science and Medicine, 131*(1), 1–9.

Graham, H., & McDermott, E. (2006). Qualitative research and the evidence base of policy: Insights from studies of teenage mothers in the UK. *Journal of Social Policy, 35*(1), 21–37.

Hosie, A. C. S. (2007). 'I hated everything about school': An examination of the relationship between dislike of school, teenage pregnancy and educational disengagement. *Social Policy and Society, 6*(3), 333–347.

Hotz, V. J., McElroy, S. W., & Sanders, S. G. (1996). The costs and consequences of teenage childbearing for mothers. *Chicago Policy Review, 64*, 55–94.

Imamura, M., Tucker, J., Hannaford, P., da Silva, M. O., Astin, M., Wyness, L., et al. (2007). Factors associated with teenage pregnancy in the European Union countries: A systematic review. *European Journal of Public Health, 17*(6), 630–636.

Kehily, M. J. (2009). *What is identity? A sociological perspective.* In: ESRC Seminar Series: The educational and social impact of new technologies on young people in Britain, London School of Economics, UK.

Kingfisher, C. P. (1996). *Women in the American welfare trap.* Philadelphia, PA: University of Pennsylvania Press.

Lottes, I. L. (2002). Sexual health policies in other industrialized countries: Are there lessons for the United States? *The Journal of Sex Research, 39*(1), 79–83.

Luttrell, W. (2003). *Pregnant bodies, fertile minds: Gender, race and the schooling of pregnant teens.* New York: Routledge.

MacDonald, R., & Marsh, J. (2005). *Disconnected youth? Growing up in Britain's poor neighbourhoods.* Basingstoke: Palgrave.

Maruna, S. (2001). *Making good: How ex-convicts reform and rebuild their lives.* Washington, DC: American Psychological Association.

McRobbie, A. (2009). *The aftermath of feminism: Gender, culture and social change*. London: Sage.

Middleton, S. (2011). 'I wouldn't change having the children - not at all'. Young women's narratives of maternal timing: What the UK's Teenage Pregnancy Strategy hasn't heard. *Sexuality Research and Social Policy, 8*, 227–238.

Ministry of Health. (2001). *Sexual and reproductive health strategy part one*. Wellington: New Zealand Ministry of Health.

Morgan, D. H. J. (2013). *Rethinking family practices*. Basingstoke: Palgrave Macmillan.

Murphy, M. (2013). Cross-national patterns of intergenerational continuities in childbearing in developed countries. *Biodemography and Social Biology, 59*(2), 101–126.

Owen, J., Higginbottom, G., Kirkham, M., Mathers, N., & Marsh, P. (2010). Young mothers from 'minoritised' backgrounds: Shakira, Lorna and Charlene. In S. Duncan, R. Edwards, & C. Alexander (Eds.), *Teenage parenthood: What's the problem?* London: Tuffnell Press.

Phoenix, A. (1991). *Young mothers*. Cambridge: Polity Press.

Rolfe, A. (2008). 'You've got to grow up when you've got a kid': Marginalized young women's accounts of motherhood. *Journal of Community and Applied Social Psychology, 18*, 299–314.

Sedgh, G., Finer, L., Bankole, A., Eilers, M., & Singh, S. (2015). Adolescent Pregnancy, birth and abortion rates across countries: Levels and recent trends. *Journal of Adolescent Health, 56*(2), 223–230.

Shea, R., Bryant, L., & Wendt, S. (2015). 'Nappy bags instead of handbags': Young motherhood and self-identity. *Journal of Sociology*. doi:10.1177/1440783315599594.

Singh, S., Darroch, J. E., & Frost, J. J. (2001). Socioeconomic disadvantage and adolescent women's sexual and reproductive behavior: The case of five developed countries. *Family Planning Perspectives, 33*(6), 251–258.

Skeggs, B. (1997). *Formations of class and gender*. London: Sage.

SmithBattle, L. (2012). Moving policies upstream to mitigate the social determinants of early childbearing. *Public Health Nursing, 29*(5), 444–454.

Social Exclusion Unit (SEU). (1999). *Teenage pregnancy*. London: Stationery Office.

Stapleton, H. (2010). *Surviving teenage motherhood; risks and realities*. Basingstoke: Palgrave Macmillan.

Thane, P., & Evans, T. (2012). *Sinners? Scroungers? Saints? Unmarried motherhood in twentieth century England*. Oxford: Oxford University Press.

Thomson, R. (2000). Dream on: The logic of sexual practice. *Journal of Youth Studies, 3*(4), 407–427.

Thomson, R., Bell, R., Holland, J., Henderson, S., McGrellis, S., & Sharpe, S. (2002). Critical moments: Choice, chance and opportunity in young people's narratives of transition. *Sociology, 36*(2), 335–354.

Thomson, R., & Holland, J. (2002). Imagining adulthood: Resources, plans and contradictions. *Gender and Education, 14*(4), 337–350.

Thomson, R., Kehily, M. J., Hadfield, L., & Sharpe, S. (2011). *Making modern mothers*. Bristol: Policy Press.

Træen, B., Stulhofer, A., & Landripet, I. (2011). Young and sexual in Norway and Croatia: Revisiting the Scandinavian versus Mediterranean gendered pattern of sexual initiation. *International Journal of Sexual Health, 23*, 196–209.

Tuffin, K., Rouch, G., & Frewin, K. (2010). Constructing adolescent fatherhood: Responsibilities and intergenerational repair. *Culture, Health and Sexuality, 12*(5), 485–498.

Tyler, I. (2013). *Revolting subjects: Social abjection and resistance in neoliberal Britain*. London: Zed Books.

Walkerdine, V., Lucey, H., & Melody, J. (2001). *Growing-up girl: Psycho-social explorations of gender and class*. London: Palgrave.

Weaver, H., Smith, G., & Kippax, S. (2005). School-based sex education policies and indicators of sexual health among young people: A comparison of the Netherlands, France, Australia and the United States. *Sex Education: Sexuality, Society and Learning, 5*(2), 171–188.

Welshman, J. (2006). *Underclass: A history of the excluded 1880–2000*. Hambledon: Continuum.

Wenham, A. (2015). 'I know I'm a good mum – No one can tell me different': Young mothers negotiating a stigmatised identity through time. *Families, Relationships and Societies*, doi:10.1332/204674315X14193466354732

Wilson, H., & Huntington, A. (2006). Deviant (M)others: The construction of teenage motherhood in contemporary discourse. *Journal of Social Policy, 35*(1), 59–76.

Index

Printed by Printforce, the Netherlands